Communications in Computer and Information Science   2386

Series Editors

Gang Li, *School of Information Technology, Deakin University, Burwood, VIC, Australia*
Joaquim Filipe, *Polytechnic Institute of Setúbal, Setúbal, Portugal*
Zhiwei Xu, *Chinese Academy of Sciences, Beijing, China*

W0235515

Rationale
The CCIS series is devoted to the publication of proceedings of computer science conferences. Its aim is to efficiently disseminate original research results in informatics in printed and electronic form. While the focus is on publication of peer-reviewed full papers presenting mature work, inclusion of reviewed short papers reporting on work in progress is welcome, too. Besides globally relevant meetings with internationally representative program committees guaranteeing a strict peer-reviewing and paper selection process, conferences run by societies or of high regional or national relevance are also considered for publication.

Topics
The topical scope of CCIS spans the entire spectrum of informatics ranging from foundational topics in the theory of computing to information and communications science and technology and a broad variety of interdisciplinary application fields.

Information for Volume Editors and Authors
Publication in CCIS is free of charge. No royalties are paid, however, we offer registered conference participants temporary free access to the online version of the conference proceedings on SpringerLink (http://link.springer.com) by means of an http referrer from the conference website and/or a number of complimentary printed copies, as specified in the official acceptance email of the event.

CCIS proceedings can be published in time for distribution at conferences or as postproceedings, and delivered in the form of printed books and/or electronically as USBs and/or e-content licenses for accessing proceedings at SpringerLink. Furthermore, CCIS proceedings are included in the CCIS electronic book series hosted in the SpringerLink digital library at http://link.springer.com/bookseries/7899. Conferences publishing in CCIS are allowed to use Online Conference Service (OCS) for managing the whole proceedings lifecycle (from submission and reviewing to preparing for publication) free of charge.

Publication process
The language of publication is exclusively English. Authors publishing in CCIS have to sign the Springer CCIS copyright transfer form, however, they are free to use their material published in CCIS for substantially changed, more elaborate subsequent publications elsewhere. For the preparation of the camera-ready papers/files, authors have to strictly adhere to the Springer CCIS Authors' Instructions and are strongly encouraged to use the CCIS LaTeX style files or templates.

Abstracting/Indexing
CCIS is abstracted/indexed in DBLP, Google Scholar, EI-Compendex, Mathematical Reviews, SCImago, Scopus. CCIS volumes are also submitted for the inclusion in ISI Proceedings.

How to start
To start the evaluation of your proposal for inclusion in the CCIS series, please send an e-mail to ccis@springer.com.

Louis Ehwerhemuepha · Mark Hoffman ·
Adam Kalawi · Terence Sanger
Editors

Pediatric and Lifespan Data Science

First International Conference, IPLDSC 2024
Anaheim, CA, USA, May 23–24, 2024
Revised Selected Papers

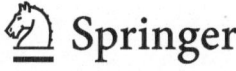 Springer

Editors
Louis Ehwerhemuepha
Children's Hospital of Orange County
Orange, CA, USA

Mark Hoffman
Children's Mercy Kansas City
Kansas City, MO, USA

Adam Kalawi
Children's Hospital of Orange County
Orange, CA, USA

Terence Sanger
Children's Hospital of Orange County
Orange, CA, USA

ISSN 1865-0929   ISSN 1865-0937 (electronic)
Communications in Computer and Information Science
ISBN 978-3-031-88345-3   ISBN 978-3-031-88346-0 (eBook)
https://doi.org/10.1007/978-3-031-88346-0

This work was supported by Children's Hospital of Orange County.

This Springer imprint is published by the registered company Springer Nature Switzerland AG
The registered company address is: Gewerbestrasse 11, 6330 Cham, Switzerland

If disposing of this product, please recycle the paper.

Preface

The proceedings of the Pediatric and Lifespan Data Science Conference showcase the top papers accepted for podium or poster presentations. This two-day event united global experts in medicine, research, and data science to tackle pressing challenges in pediatric and lifespan research. Health evolves with shifting risk factors, symptoms, and clinical interventions throughout our lives. The conference focused on the unique requirements and technological tools needed to analyze data across all life stages, from childhood to advanced age.

Thirty abstracts were submitted from which 8 were selected and invited to submit for publication as full papers in the conference proceedings. Additionally two conference narratives were invited for submission, these are descriptions of the panel sessions and they are included in the back matter of this volume. Consequently, there were a total of 10 submissions selected for inclusion in this volume out of 32 possible entries.

Louis Ehwerhemuepha
Mark Hoffman
Adam Kalawi
Terence Sanger

Organization

Program Committee Chairs

Ehwerhemuepha, Louis   Children's Hospital of Orange County, California, USA

Hoffman, Mark   Children's Mercy, Kansas City, USA

Kalawi, Adam   Children's Hospital of Orange County, California, USA

Sanger, Terence   Children's Hospital of Orange County, California, USA

Program Committee Members

Devin, Joan   Rotunda Hospital, Ireland

Ehwerhemuepha, Louis   Children's Hospital of Orange County, California, USA

Hoffman, Mark   Children's Mercy Kansas City, USA

Kalawi, Adam   Children's Hospital of Orange County, California, USA

Kassani, Peyman   Children's Hospital of Orange County, California, USA

Nagarajan, Radha   Children's Hospital of Orange County, California, USA

Rasouli, Mahkameh   University of California, Irvine, USA

Wayland, Jeremy   Institute of AI for Health, Helmholtz Munich, Germany

Reviewers

Aguilar, Ricardo   Children's Hospital of Orange County, California, USA

Devin, Joan   Rotunda Hospital, Ireland

Ehwerhemuepha, Louis   Children's Hospital of Orange County, California, USA

Grisel Todorov, Nikolay   Chapman University, USA

Hoffman, Mark   Children's Mercy Kansas City, USA

Kalawi, Adam	Children's Hospital of Orange County, California, USA
Kassani, Peyman	Children's Hospital of Orange County, California, USA
Martel, Steven	Children's Hospital of Orange County, California, USA
Nagarajan, Radha	Children's Hospital of Orange County, California, USA
Rasouli, Mahkameh	University of California, Irvine, USA
Thompson, Jeffrey	University of Kansas Medical Center, USA
Wayland, Jeremy	Institute of AI for Health, Helmholtz Munich, Germany
Yaghmaei, Ehsan	Chapman University, USA

Contents

tabular data, are limited in their ability to distill complex dynamics among physicians. Graph representations and tools from network analysis have thus been adopted in the literature to provide more sophisticated models for care delivery [2–4, 6, 6, 13, 15, 20, 23, 26, 27, 29, 30], permitting an understanding of the data both on the local and the global level. Increased access to medical claims data has placed an emphasis on analyzing *Physician Referral Networks*, which encode patient sharing between physicians across different regions in the United States. Physician Referral Networks are typically modeled using administrative claims data (often from Medicare) to map patient-flow patterns, elucidating more complex dynamics that underpin local care delivery. Their study has proved fruitful for enhancing care coordination, reducing costs, improving patient outcomes, and understanding social determinants of health [11, 16, 18, 25].

Our work aims to introduce novel foundational tools to the study of Physician Referral Networks. In particular, we focus on curvature-based measures for capturing structural properties of a graph. Ricci curvature, a well-known concept in differential geometry, has recently gained traction for various applications in the field of machine learning [9, 10, 35]. In fact, *positive* Ricci curvature in a network was shown to correspond to regions of high connectivity—which, in the context of care delivery, could represent tighter-knit groups with the capacity for better coordination and communication. *Negative* curvature, by contrast, is known to capture information bottlenecks in message-passing neural networks [37], and has the potential to indicate less robust regions in a referral network that are prone to information loss, miscommunication, and potentially lower standards of care.

In addition to strong theoretical foundations and promising interpretations in the context of care delivery, Ricci curvature measures also stand out against standard network descriptors (e.g., assortativity, centrality, clustering coefficients) due to their ability to precisely describe the structure of a network and their flexibility in easily switching between edge-level, node-level, or network-level aggregations to suit the analysis at hand [36]. Thus, we aim to bolster foundational analysis of Physician Referral Networks with the following **key contributions**:

1. We introduce Ricci curvature-based measures as novel structural features for characterizing Physician Referral Networks.
2. We perform initial analyses using these measures to study healthcare delivery across diverse U.S. regions.
3. We develop apparent, an open-access tool that empowers researchers studying U.S. healthcare delivery by offering an interactive platform to explore referral network features and their correlations with local census data, healthcare effectiveness, and patient outcomes.

2   Background

Research on Physician Referral Networks has evolved significantly, transitioning from small-scale empirical studies to large-scale analyses enabled by the advent

Characterizing Physician Referral Networks with Ricci Curvature

Jeremy Wayland[1,2](✉)📧 , Russell J. Funk[4]📧 , and Bastian Rieck[1,2,3]📧

[1] Information and Technology, Technical University of Munich School of Computation, Arcisstraße 21, 80333 Munich, Germany
bastian.grossenbacher@unifr.ch
[2] Institute of AI for Health, Helmholtz Munich, Ingolstädter Landstraße 1, 85764 Oberschleißheim, Germany
jeremydon.wayland@helmholtz-munich.de
[3] Department of Informatics, University of Fribourg, Boulevard de Pérolles 90, Fribourg, Fribourg 1700, Switzerland
[4] Carlson School of Management, University of Minnesota, 321 19th Avenue South, Minneapolis, MN 55455, USA
rfunk@umn.edu

Abstract. Identifying (a) systemic barriers to quality healthcare access and (b) key indicators of care efficacy in the United States remains a significant challenge. To improve our understanding of regional disparities in care delivery, we introduce a novel application of curvature, a geometrical-topological property of networks, to Physician Referral Networks. Our initial findings reveal that *Forman-Ricci* and *Ollivier-Ricci* curvature measures, which are known for their expressive power in characterizing network structure, offer promising indicators for detecting variations in healthcare efficacy while capturing a range of significant regional demographic features. We also present apparent, an open-source tool that leverages Ricci curvature and other network features to examine correlations between regional Physician Referral Networks structure, local census data, healthcare effectiveness, and patient outcomes.

1 Introduction

In the rapidly evolving field of healthcare management, the analysis of medical claims data has become an essential component for improving the quality and equity of healthcare services. The nature of care delivery in the United States is heavily influenced by its fragmentation—care is often spread across multiple disconnected providers (e.g., primary-care physicians, specialists). Settings with greater care fragmentation have been shown to inhibit effective communication and coordination between care team members, thus contributing to higher costs and lower quality of care [1,7,14,22,34].

Despite the well-understood impacts of fragmentation, there are still few quantitative tools that can capture the mechanisms of care delivery networks at scale [15]. Standard analyses of local infrastructure features, often executed using

ⓒ The Author(s) 2025
L. Ehwerhemuepha et al. (Eds.): IPLDSC 2024, CCIS 2386, pp. 1–16, 2025.
https://doi.org/10.1007/978-3-031-88346-0_1

of large-scale data access [5,15,21,25,31,32]. This progression has expanded the scope and depth of understanding regarding the structure and dynamics of care delivery networks. Early empirical studies, despite being constrained to individual care delivery networks and often involving only several thousand physicians, provided essential insights into the conceptualization of Physician Referral Networks and their ability to characterize healthcare delivery [11,25]. Recently, the growing availability of large-scale administrative data, particularly from electronic medical records and insurance claims, has allowed for more robust studies on Physician Referral Networks across the country. This work examines quantitative network properties to glean insights on care coordination, utilization, and cost, as well as relationships between network structure and economic/clinical outcomes [13,16,20,30].

However, significant challenges remain in effectively and efficiently extracting relevant features from these complex data structures. Key obstacles include the high dimensionality of network data, the computational complexity of analyzing large-scale networks, and the difficulty in interpreting network measures in clinical contexts. This creates a crucial need for new analytical approaches. Bridging the gap between foundational theory and contemporary measurement has already shown promising results for care delivery analysis [15,23,29]. By introducing Ricci curvature, we aim to further expand this frontier, leveraging a rich mathematical tradition in differential geometry to enhance our collective interpretations when evaluating these intricate healthcare systems.

3 Data Description

We analyze Medicare claims data in the United States from 2014–2017, consisting of 663,541 total physicians, with approximately 10,000,000 patient-sharing records per year across 3404 Hospital Service Areas (HSAs). These data were made publicly available by CareSet a healthcare data consultancy, in collaboration with the Center for Medicare and Medicaid Services (CMS), the U.S. government agency that administers Medicare, and have been widely used in prior research on physician networks [12,17,19,24]. As outlined in Table 1, we supplement physician interactions with data from several sources including basic data on the physicians included in our networks (e.g., practice locations, specialty types) from the National Plan and Provider Enumeration System (NPPES) as well as metrics on local healthcare quality and spending from the Dartmouth Institute for Health Policy and Clinical Practice.

Data Format. The data are provided in the form of edge lists (i.e., pairs of physicians). The nodes correspond to physicians, who are assigned unique, numerical codes corresponding to their National Provider Identifiers (NPIs). Physicians are linked by an edge when they treat the same patients within a specified timeframe. The strength of this connection is measured by the number of patients they have in common. For instance, if Physician A treated 30 patients in one week, and 12 of those patients were seen by Physician B the following week,

Table 1. Data Release Summary. We provide an overview of the tables that comprise our original database, along with high level descriptions of their features and relevance for characterizing local Physician Referral Networks. Up-to-date table structure, data summaries, and feature descriptions will be maintained within our prototype, apparent.

Table Name	Description
referral_network_features	Features of Physician Referral Networks by HSA and year, including network metrics such as assortativity, clustering, density, Forman-Ricci, and Ollivier-Ricci Curvatures. These metrics provide insights into the structure and connectivity of local physician networks.
hedis_measures	Contains Healthcare Effectiveness Data and Information Set (HEDIS) measures by Health Service Area (HSA) and year, including various diabetes and mammography metrics segmented by race. These measures are crucial for evaluating healthcare quality and outcomes across different regions and demographics.
hospital_atlas_data	Includes information about hospitals such as provider details, location, teaching status, and bed counts. This data is essential for understanding the distribution and capacity of healthcare facilities within local networks.
population_census	Provides demographic data by HSA and year, including population counts by race, median household income, employment, and education levels. This demographic information is important for analyzing the socioeconomic context of healthcare networks.
post_discharge_records	Contains post-discharge outcomes for various conditions by HSA and year, such as readmission rates and follow-up care. This data helps assess the effectiveness of patient transitions from hospital to home care.
standard_pricing	Includes standard pricing and payments for various medical services by HSA and year. Understanding pricing variations is important for economic analyses of healthcare delivery and cost efficiency.
local_physician_interactions	Contains Medicare claims data by year and HSA, detailing interactions between physicians (identified by NPI numbers). This data is the sole generator for the Physician Referral Networks.

we would establish a connection between A and B with a strength value of 12. We exclude from our analysis organizational providers (e.g., hospitals, clinics) such that all nodes in our networks correspond to individuals. We also limit the networks to include only physicians who are likely to be directly involved with patient care (e.g., we remove radiologists). The list of included physicians was developed in consultation with a team of clinicians.

Location Information. Healthcare delivery in the United States tends to be highly localized, with substantial variation in both healthcare practices and outcomes across regions. To capture this variation, we map physician networks separately by region, focusing on Hospital Service Areas (HSAs; as defined by the Dartmouth Atlas). HSAs have been widely used in prior research on healthcare delivery and are designed to correspond roughly to local markets for hospital services. We position physicians within HSAs by geocoding their practice locations; as such, our network maps consist of shared patients among the physicians practicing within a particular HSA. Finally, we study networks separately by year, for each of the four years in our study window, recognizing that the structure of Physician Referral Networks may change over time.

Selection Criteria. To protect patient privacy and comply with CMS regulations, we only include physician pairs in our data if they shared at least 11 patients within a specific time period [8]. While this thresholding approach necessarily results in some data loss, previous research suggests that connections between physicians based on few shared patients are often not considered significant by the physicians themselves [5]. The most meaningful professional relationships typically involve a higher number of shared patients and align more closely with survey data. Therefore, this required minimum threshold is actually beneficial, as it likely produces networks that more accurately reflect real-world professional relationships.

4   Methods

4.1   Building Physician Referral Networks

Similar to social or biological networks, we can model Physician Referral Networks as graphs. A graph $G := (V, E)$ consists of a set of nodes V that model the objects of interest in a system and a set of edges E that encode relationships between the nodes. In the context of care delivery, nodes often represent healthcare providers, such as physicians, and edges can represent patient-sharing relationships or referrals between these providers.

Our goal is to capture patient flow within an HSA during the course of a year. Each provider in the HSA becomes a node in the graph, and edges are assigned between physicians when a sufficient number of patients are shared via referrals. We provide some real examples in Fig. 1 that arise from HSAs in different regions of the country (Southern California vs. Atlanta). Our graph representations are built directly from the `local_physician_interactions` table (see Table 1).

4.2   Ricci Curvature

Ricci curvature is a fundamental concept situated at the intersection of differential geometry and topology that has recently emerged as a powerful tool in graph machine learning [9,10,28,33,37]. Curvature measures for graphs offer a concise yet comprehensive way to represent and analyze structural features of networks, serving as a lens for measuring local "cohesiveness." Among the various curvature constructions, our work focuses on two specific types of Ricci curvature: *Forman-Ricci* and *Ollivier-Ricci*. Both of these measures evaluate how the volume growth of a network deviates from that of a "model" Euclidean space, providing nuanced insights into network structure. This is achieved by capturing the similarity between neighborhoods of nodes. For some token examples of positively- and negatively-curved Physician Referral Networks, see Fig. 2

Similar to their continuous counterparts, discrete network curvature measures permit the following interpretations:

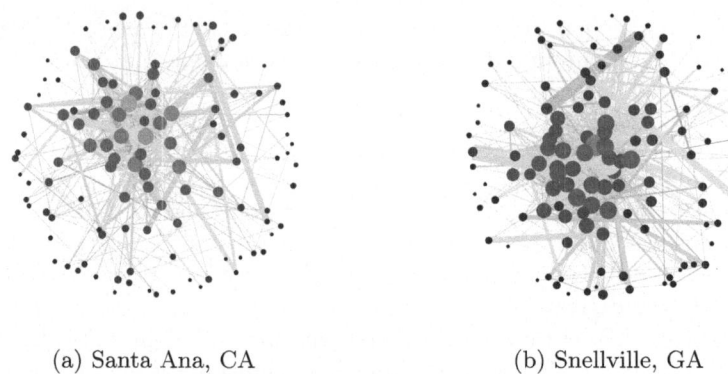

(a) Santa Ana, CA   (b) Snellville, GA

Fig. 1. Visualizing Physician Referral Networks. Above, we visualize networks from regions with known differences in care delivery. Figure 1a shows a referral network from Santa Ana, California, exhibiting a higher quality of care, while Fig. 1b comes from Snellville, Georgia. As made available in apparent, we combine traditional network features with Ricci Curvature to elucidate the structural properties of care delivery in each region: Nodes are sized and colored by centrality and degree while edges are sized and colored by number of referrals and κ_{OR}, respectively. *Interpretation:* Larger yellow nodes are physicians that play a prominent role in regional care delivery by dictating patient flow. Blue-gray edges (negative curvature) are potential bottlenecks for patients finding the best provider, while orange edges (positive curvature) indicate strong communication between physicians and well-established patient flow.

- **Positive curvature** indicates configurations with overlapping neighborhoods, such as cliques, where nodes are well-connected.
- **Zero or low curvature** is associated with grid-like structures, where connectivity is more uniform but less dense.
- **Negative curvature** often appears in tree-like formations, where nodes have fewer overlapping neighbors and connectivity is more sparse.

In comparison with standard network descriptors such as assortativity, centrality, and clustering coefficients, Ricci curvature offers greater *expressiveness*—meaning these measures are more effective at distinguishing between non-isomorphic graphs [36]. Additionally, curvature measures can be aggregated to provide insights at different levels (edge, node, or network) allowing for a detailed analysis of specific physicians, their relationships, or a summary comparison between different networks. We hope to inspire practitioners and researchers interested in healthcare management and delivery systems to incorporate curvature-based measures into their network analysis pipelines.

Forman-Ricci Curvature. Forman-Ricci Curvature (FRC) is a discrete curvature measure for edges in a network based on local connectivity. In the context of physician networks, FRC measure provides an efficient, albeit less expressive, measure for evaluating the collaboration patterns among physicians. The formula for Forman-Ricci Curvature between two connected nodes i and j is given by:

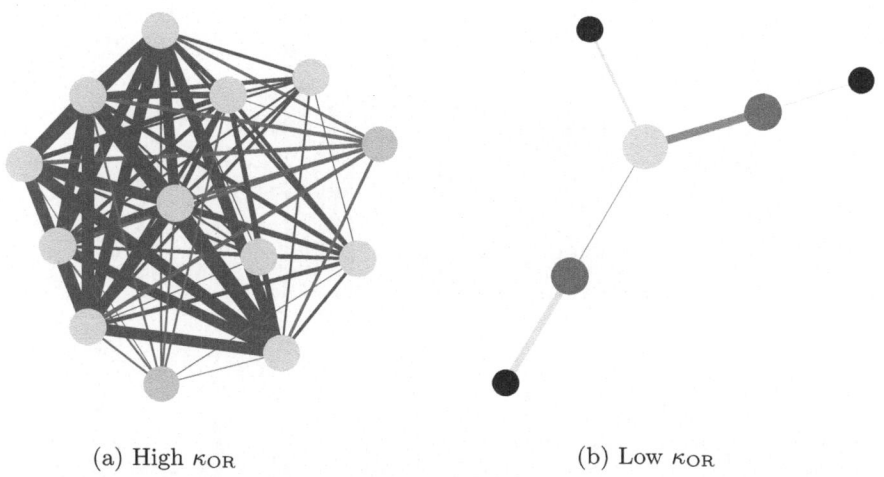

(a) High κ_{OR} (b) Low κ_{OR}

Fig. 2. Ollivier-Ricci Curvature for Physician Referral Networks. In care delivery networks, *positive* Ricci curvature, as seen in Fig. 2a, can highlight regions with high connectivity and well-coordinated groups, potentially indicating better communication and care coordination. Conversely, *negative* curvature, seen in Fig. 2b, can signal areas prone to information bottlenecks, which might lead to communication issues and lower care quality.

$$\kappa_{\mathrm{FR}}(i,j) := 4 - d_i - d_j + 3|\#_\Delta| \tag{1}$$

Here, d_i and d_j denote the degrees of nodes i and j, respectively, and $|\#_\Delta|$ represents the number of triangles (i.e., 3-cliques) that include the edge (i,j). In Physician Referral Networks, d_i and d_j correspond to the number of direct connections (referrals) each physician has, while $|\#_\Delta|$ indicates the number of mutual connections between the two physicians. A higher FRC value suggests a stronger collaborative relationship, characterized by more mutual connections and shared professional interactions. In general FRC values are unbounded— in large networks edges can take large positive or large negative values (see Fig. 4). As an intuitive example for an edge with very *negative* κ_{FR}, imagine two communities modeled as fully connected graphs that are connected by a single edge. Each community can be made to have arbitrarily large degrees (d_i, d_j in Eq. (1)), but the edge between them cannot have mutual connections (i.e., $|\#_\Delta| = 0$).

Ollivier-Ricci Curvature. Ollivier-Ricci Curvature (ORC) is a more expressive measure than FRC that quantifies the curvature of edges in a graph by comparing the neighborhoods of the nodes connected by the edge. Rather than counting triangles, a more sophisticated comparison is achieved using methods from optimal-transport theory; specifically, the Wasserstein distance (also known as Earth Mover's distance) between the probability distributions associated with node neighborhoods is evaluated. The formula for Ollivier-Ricci Cur-

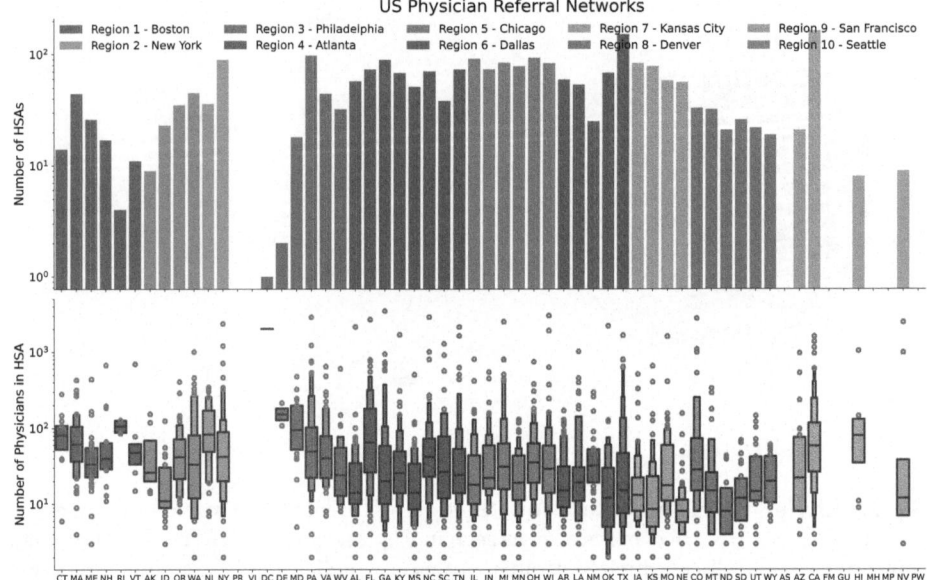

Fig. 3. Regional Distribution of Physician Referral Networks. Here we visualize the distribution of Physician Referral Networks in 2017 (one per Health Service Area, HSA) alongside physician counts (nodes) by state, color-coded by region. This figure highlights the relative *size* and *density* of Physician Referral Networks and establishes a baseline for structural differences in care coordination across the United States.

vature between two connected nodes i and j is given by:

$$\kappa_{\mathrm{OR}}(i,j) := 1 - \frac{1}{d_G(i,j)} W_1(\mu_i, \mu_j) \tag{2}$$

Here, $d_G(i,j)$ represents the shortest path distance between nodes i and j in the graph, and $W_1(\mu_i, \mu_j)$ denotes the Wasserstein distance between the probability measures μ_i and μ_j, which are defined over the neighborhoods of nodes i and j, respectively.[1]

In the context of physician networks, μ_i and μ_j can be understood as distributions of patient referrals or collaborations within the neighborhoods of physicians i and j. A higher ORC value indicates that the neighborhoods of the two nodes are more similar, suggesting more cohesive collaboration patterns. For extreme examples or positive and negative ORC, see Fig. 2. Despite its enhanced expressiveness in capturing distinct structural properties of networks, even for challenging tasks such as distinguishing Strongly-Regular and Rook-Shrikhande graphs [36], ORC is computationally expensive for very large graphs. In contrast, FRC offers a more scalable alternative. If FRC can capture meaningful signals, it provides a practical advantage as it can be computed efficiently, even for the largest Physician Referral Networks in the United States.

---

[1] Our computations use uniform probability distributions.

5   Results

Our interactive database contains information on approximately 13,500 physician networks (bounded by HSAs), sourced over the years 2014–2017. Along with approximately 20 network descriptors, including statistics for network assortativity, clustering coefficients, density, centrality, Forman-Ricci Curvature, and Ollivier-Ricci Curvature, we also provide infrastructure for querying rich metadata for these networks. Table 1 provides a summary of the available tables and their basic descriptions.

As a preliminary case study that highlights the utility of our proposed techniques, we perform an analysis of the regional referral networks. More specifically, we explore approximately 4000 HSAs with available referral data in 2017. Figure 3 describes the distribution of Physician Referral Networks by state, split into 10 larger regions often used for healthcare analysis, while also depicting the distribution of network sizes.

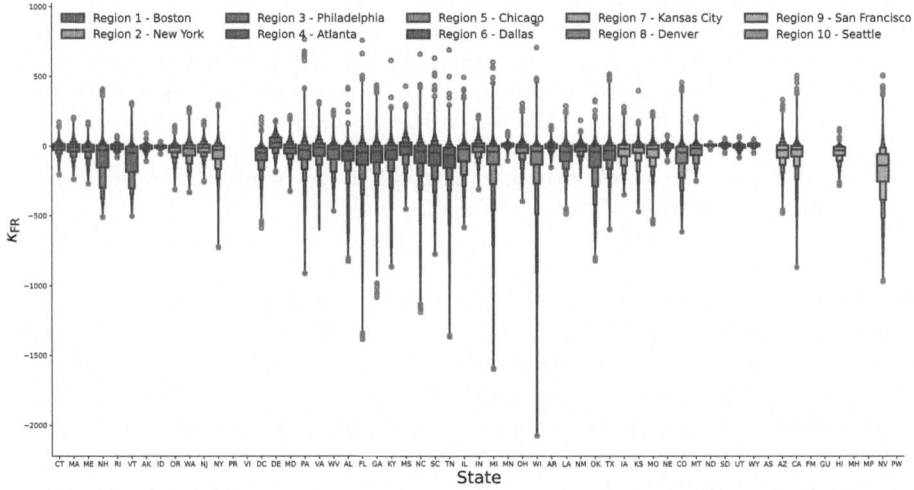

Fig. 4. Regional Distribution of Forman-Ricci Curvature. This figure displays a wide range of inter- and intra-regional differences in care delivery structure as measured by κ_{FR}. We plot curvature values for each edge (provider connection) for all 2017 Physician Referral Networks.

Additionally, we provide distributions of Forman-Ricci and Ollivier-Ricci Curvature values for network edges, grouped by state and region in Figs. 4 and 5. As we observe from the distribution, ORC values are constrained to a much tighter range, with the most negatively curved edges in our distribution approaching a value of -2, while all edge curvatures are bounded above by $+1$. In comparison, Forman-Ricci, due to its dependence on node degree and the number of triangles, can produce very large curvature values, both negative

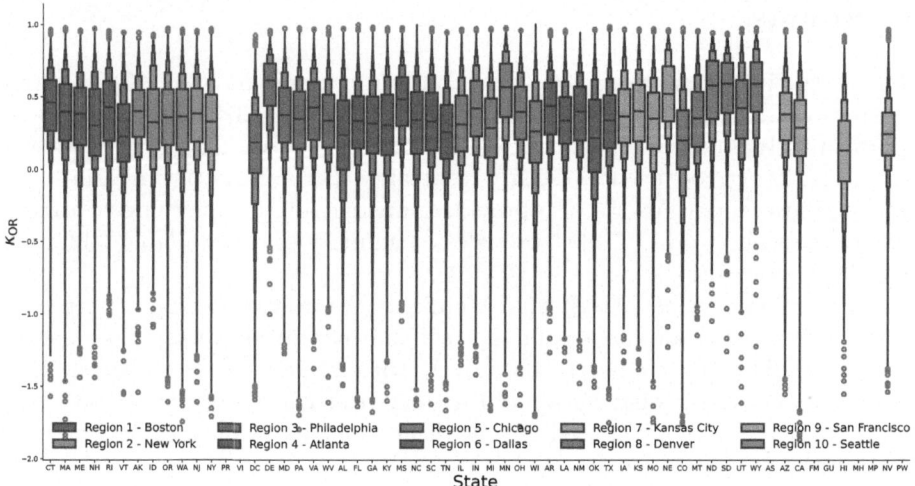

Fig. 5. Regional Distribution of Ollivier-Ricci Curvature This figure displays the regional differences in care delivery structure as measured by κ_{OR}. We plot curvature values for each edge (provider connection) for all 2017 Physician Referral Networks, separated by state and colored by region. In comparison with κ_{FR} (see Fig. 4), we see much smaller variance in κ_{OR} values which is expected based on their construction in Eq. (1) and Eq. (2). Although κ_{OR} is known to be a more *expressive* measure for capturing fine-grained network structure, although it can be much more expensive to compute for large networks.

and positive. Given the known trade-off between locality, expressivity, and efficiency between Forman-Ricci and Ollivier-Ricci Curvature [35], further analysis is required to understand which descriptors are most useful for specific healthcare management tasks. Despite clear agreement between various classical network science features (e.g., Fig. 6), Ricci curvature measures are known to be much more expressive in capturing network structure. Moreover, there is precedence for alleviating bottlenecks in graph neural networks by rewiring negatively curved edges in a network [37]. This provides a novel way to potentially "rewire" care delivery networks using these measures in order to improve healthcare quality in regions that suffer from care fragmentation.

As part of our preliminary analysis, we compared Forman-Ricci Curvature with various population statistics, including Medicare enrollment, total mortality, and the proportion of non-white populations. As seen in Fig. 7, our findings reveal that large networks exhibiting low average curvature-indicating many potential bottlenecks in care delivery-correlate with high Medicare enrollment, elevated mortality rates, and higher proportions of Black and Hispanic populations. These results (which can be reproduced interactively with apparent) suggest that negatively curved edges are indicative of structural properties in physician networks commonly found in less affluent HSAs.

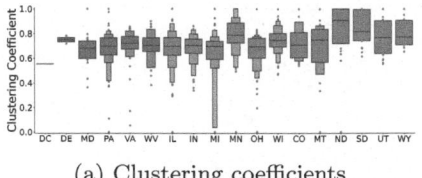

(a) Clustering coefficients

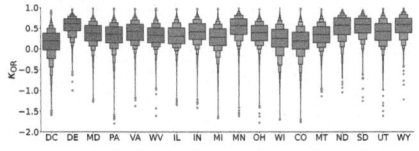

(b) Ollivier-Ricci Edge Curvatures

Fig. 6. Comparing Standard Network Features and Ricci Curvature. For a select set of states in the Philadelphia (green), Chicago (purple), and Denver (gray) HSA regions, we visualize distributions of *clustering coefficients* (CC) in comparison to κ_{OR}. These are different measures (with clearly different distributions) for capturing connectivity in a network. In the context of care delivery positive CC and κ_{OR} values together could indicate high-functioning subregions of a Physician Referral Network (Color figure online).

Our analysis demonstrates significant variation in curvature across different regions, effectively capturing disparities in network structures. The observed negative curvature in areas with higher minority populations highlights the potential for developing recommendation technologies that could enhance patient flow and improve care accessibility with minimal intervention. However, much remains to be explored, and we believe that the tools and data used in this study provide promising future avenues to better understand and address the complexities within Physician Referral Networks.

6   Discussion

6.1   Significance for Healthcare Management

Our open-source infrastructure enables network analysis on medical claims data. This opens the door for exciting advancements in healthcare management. By leveraging network analysis techniques, we can uncover intricate patterns and relationships within healthcare delivery systems that were previously hidden. This is crucial for several reasons:

- **Optimization of Care Coordination.** Understanding referral patterns and physician collaborations can help identify inefficiencies and bottlenecks in patient flow, leading to more effective care coordination.
- **Resource Allocation.** Network analysis can inform strategic decisions regarding resource distribution, ensuring that healthcare facilities and services are optimally positioned to meet patient needs.
- **Policy Development.** Insights from network structures can guide policy-makers in developing initiatives that foster more robust and integrated healthcare systems.

By collecting and combining standard network features, local census data, healthcare efficacy, treatment outcomes, along with Ricci curvature, we hope to empower researchers in healthcare management to make expedited progress on unraveling and correcting care fragmentation across the United States.

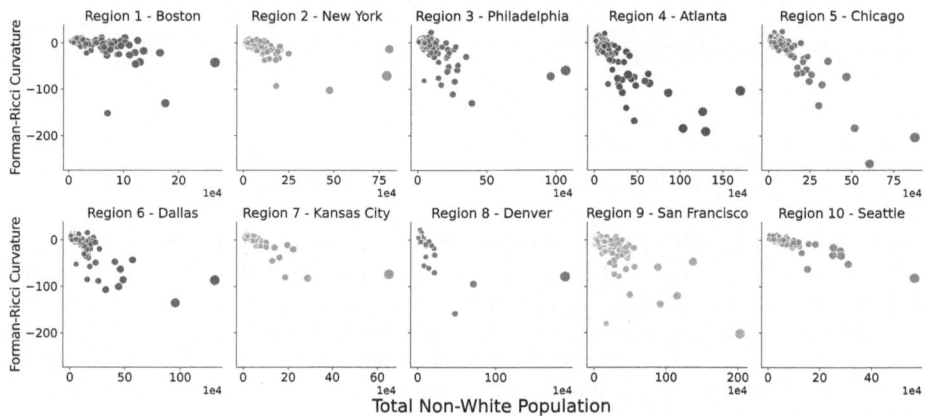

Fig. 7. Ricci-Curvature vs. Non-White Population. Across different healthcare regions, we visualize the correlation between average Forman-Ricci (κ_{FR}) curvature and total non-white population (node sizes correspond to network size). Despite clear inter-regional variation, there is consistent correlation between high non-white population in large networks with highly negative average curvature. Although these results are preliminary, they are consistent with prior work suggesting that Physician Referral Networks serving historically marginalized populations exhibit systematically less robust connectivity and therefore are less equipped to deliver high quality, low cost care.

6.2   The Promise of Ricci Curvature

Ricci curvature measures for characterizing edges in a network have proven to be expressive both in terms of structural analysis of networks and identifying bottlenecks in information flow. Our work is the first to bring these geometric measures into the field of healthcare management. In particular, we compute and openly distribute our results of computing *Ollivier-Ricci* and *Forman-Ricci* curvature, and present promising results that indicate that bottlenecks in Physician Referral Networks (as measured by curvature) correlate highly with metadata associated with healthcare systems that are known to receive a lower standard of care.

6.3   Exploration Prototype

To further the impact of our research, we provide an open-access dataset and analysis suite, apparent that combines medical claims data with various demographic and socioeconomic factors. This provides access to network features and abundant metadata, along with prototypes for exploring/visualizing user queries. Additionally, we provide a Python repository[2] that allows users to interact directly with the dataset. This repository supports building, customizing, and reproducing Physician Referral Networks and associated structural features, as

---

[2] Our codebase is maintained at: https://github.com/aidos-lab/apparent.

well as visualizing networks and feature distributions. By offering access to curvature features and other network metrics, we empower both technical and nontechnical researchers to explore the data, fostering a collaborative environment for discovering new insights.

6.4   Limitations

While our approach offers many advantages, there are several limitations to consider:

- **Computational Tractability.** Calculating κ_{OR} on massive networks is computationally intensive, limiting its scalability. Thus, we recommend users to prioritize κ_{FR} for studying large scale Physician Referral Networks.
- **Network Specifications.** We only build and analyze unweighted, undirected networks, which may overlook the complexities of real-world healthcare interactions. We hope to extend our analyses to more complex network constructions in the future.
- **Feature Completeness.** Our prototype may lack some critical features necessary for a comprehensive understanding of healthcare management. This prototype serves as a foundation for future enhancements, and can easily be updated as necessary.

6.5   Future Work

Looking ahead, we aim to expand our research in several key areas:

- **Network Evolution.** Studying how healthcare networks evolve over time to identify trends and predict future changes.
- **Thorough Data Analysis.** Conducting a more detailed analysis of existing data to derive actionable insights that can influence policy and management decisions.
- **Regional Characteristics.** Understanding the distinctive features of regional healthcare networks and how they relate to specific policies and practices.
- **Edge Prediction.** Developing methods for predicting new referrals that could alleviate bottlenecks in patient flow, utilizing negative curvature as a predictive metric.

We hope apparent will serve as a valuable resource, enabling researchers and practitioners to explore networks, network features (including curvature), and various other metadata, inspiring deeper investigations and support data-driven decision-making in healthcare management.

Acknowledgements. We would like to acknowledge the authors and developers of the Datasette package, whose work has been instrumental in the development of our open-source prototype. Their tool has enabled us to efficiently manage, explore, and visualize our dataset, significantly enhancing our ability to analyze and share our findings. We also thank the members of the CARE-CONNECT team, as well as Corinna Coupette for her valuable insights during the early stages of the project and her assistance in creating visualizations, and Katharina Limbeck for her helpful review of the final manuscript. Research reported in this publication was supported by the National Heart, Lung, And Blood Institute of the National Institutes of Health under Award Number R01HL167816. The content is solely the responsibility of the authors and does not necessarily represent the official views of the National Institutes of Health. B.R. is partially supported by the Bavarian state government with funds from the *Hightech Agenda Bavaria*.

References

1. Agha, L., Frandsen, B., Rebitzer, J.B.: Fragmented division of labor and healthcare costs: Evidence from moves across regions. J. Public Econ. **169**, 144–159 (2019)
2. An, C., O'Malley, A.J., Rockmore, D.N., Stock, C.D.: Analysis of the US patient referral network. Stat. Med. **37**(5), 847–866 (2018)
3. An, C., O'Malley, A.J., Rockmore, D.N.: Referral paths in the US physician network. Appli. Netw. Sci. **3**, 1–24 (2018)
4. Barnett, M.L., Christakis, N.A., O'Malley, J., Onnela, J.P., Keating, N.L., Landon, B.E.: Physician patient-sharing networks and the cost and intensity of care in US hospitals. Med. Care **50**(2), 152–160 (2012)
5. Barnett, M.L., Landon, B.E., O'malley, A.J., Keating, N.L., Christakis, N.A.: Mapping physician networks with self-reported and administrative data. Health Serv. Res. **46**(5), 1592–1609 (2011)
6. Casalino, L.P., et al.: Physician networks and ambulatory care-sensitive admissions. Med. Care **53**(6), 534–541 (2015)
7. Cebul, R.D., Rebitzer, J.B., Taylor, L.J., Votruba, M.E.: Organizational fragmentation and care quality in the US healthcare system. J. Econ. Perspect. **22**(4), 93–113 (2008)
8. Centers for Medicare & Medicaid Services: Medicaid program; establishing minimum standards for medicaid managed care plans. Federal Register (May 2024), docket Number: CMS-2439-F, RIN: 0938-AU99
9. Coupette, C., Dalleiger, S., Rieck, B.: Ollivier-Ricci curvature for hypergraphs: A unified framework. In: International Conference on Learning Representations (2023). https://openreview.net/forum?id=sPCKNl5qDps
10. Devriendt, K., Lambiotte, R.: Discrete curvature on graphs from the effective resistance. J. Phys. Complexity **3**(2), 025008 (2022). https://doi.org/10.1088/2632-072x/ac730d
11. DuGoff, E.H., Fernandes-Taylor, S., Weissman, G.E., Huntley, J.H., Pollack, C.E.: A scoping review of patient-sharing network studies using administrative data. Trans. Behav. Med. **8**(4), 598–625 (2018). https://doi.org/10.1093/tbm/ibx015
12. Everson, J., Adler-Milstein, J.: Electronic connectivity among US hospitals treating shared patients. Med. Care **60**(12), 880–887 (2022)
13. Everson, J., et al.: Repeated, close physician coronary artery bypass grafting teams associated with greater teamwork. Health Serv. Res. **53**(2), 1025–1041 (2018)
14. Frandsen, B.R., Joynt, K.E., Rebitzer, J.B., Jha, A.K.: Care fragmentation, quality, and costs among chronically ill patients. Am. J. Managed Care **21**(5), 355–362 (2015)

15. Funk, R.J., Owen-Smith, J., Kaufman, S.A., Nallamothu, B.K., Hollingsworth, J.M.: Association of informal clinical integration of physicians with cardiac surgery payments. JAMA Surg. **153**(5), 446–453 (2018)
16. Gandré, C., Beauguitte, L., Lolivier, A., Coldefy, M.: Care coordination for severe mental health disorders: an analysis of healthcare provider patient-sharing networks and their association with quality of care in a French region. BMC Health Serv. Res. **20**(1), 548 (2020). https://doi.org/10.1186/s12913-020-05173-x
17. Gebhart, T., Fu, X., Funk, R.J.: Go with the flow? a large-scale analysis of health care delivery networks in the United States using Hodge theory. In: IEEE International Conference on Big Data, pp. 3812–3823 (2021)
18. Ghomrawi, H., Funk, R.J., Parks, M.L., Owen-Smith, J., Hollingsworth, J.M.: Physician referral patterns and racial disparities in total hip replacement: a network analysis approach. PLoS ONE **13**(2), e0193014 (2018). https://doi.org/10.1371/journal.pone.0193014
19. Graves, J.A., et al.: Physician patient sharing relationships within insurance plan networks. Health Serv. Res. **58**(5), 1056–1065 (2023)
20. Hollingsworth, J.M., et al.: Differences between physician social networks for cardiac surgery serving communities with high versus low proportions of black residents. Med. Care **53**(2), 160–167 (2015)
21. Javalgi, R., Joseph, W.B., Gombeski Jr., W.R., Lester, J.A.: How physicians make referrals. J. Health Care Market. **13**(2) (1993)
22. Juo, Y.Y., Sanaiha, Y., Khrucharoen, U., Chang, B.H., Dutson, E., Benharash, P.: Care fragmentation is associated with increased short-term mortality during postoperative readmissions: a systematic review and meta-analysis. Surgery **165**(3), 501–509 (2019)
23. Kim, D., Funk, R.J., Yan, P., Nallamothu, B.K., Zaheer, A., Hollingsworth, J.M.: Informal clinical integration in medicare accountable care organizations and mortality following coronary artery bypass graft surgery. Med. Care **57**(3), 194–201 (2019)
24. Kim, K.D., Funk, R.J., Zaheer, A.: Structure in context: a morphological view of whole network performance. Soc. Netw. **72**, 165–182 (2023)
25. Landon, B.E., et al.: Variation in patient-sharing networks of physicians across the United States. JAMA **308**(3), 265–273 (2012). https://doi.org/10.1001/jama.2012.7615
26. Landon, B.E., Keating, N.L., Onnela, J.P., Zaslavsky, A.M., Christakis, N.A., O'Malley, A.J.: Patient-sharing networks of physicians and health care utilization and spending among Medicare beneficiaries. JAMA Intern. Med. **178**(1), 66–73 (2018)
27. Matthews, L.J., et al.: Within-physician differences in patient sharing between primary care physicians and cardiologists who treat white and black patients with heart disease. J. Am. Heart Assoc. **12**(22), e030653 (2023)
28. Ni, C.C., Lin, Y.Y., Gao, J., Gu, X.D., Saucan, E.: Ricci Curvature of the Internet Topology (2015). https://doi.org/10.48550/arXiv.1501.04138
29. Pollack, C.E., Weissman, G.E., Lemke, K.W., Hussey, P.S., Weiner, J.P.: Patient sharing among physicians and costs of care: a network analytic approach to care coordination using claims data. J. Gen. Intern. Med. **28**, 459–465 (2013)
30. Popescu, I., et al.: The segregation of physician networks providing care to black and white patients with heart disease: concepts, measures, and empirical evaluation. Soc. Sci. Med. **343**, 116511 (2024)
31. Shortell, S.M.: Determinants of physician referral rates: an exchange theory approach. Med. Care **12**(1), 13–31 (1974)

32. Shortell, S.M., Anderson, O.W.: The physician referral process: a theoretical perspective. Health Serv. Res. **6**(1), 39 (1971)
33. Sia, J., Jonckheere, E., Bogdan, P.: Ollivier-ricci curvature-based method to community detection in complex networks. Sci. Rep. **9**, 9800 (2019). https://doi.org/10.1038/s41598-019-46079-x
34. Snow, K., Galaviz, K., Turbow, S.: Patient outcomes following interhospital care fragmentation: a systematic review. J. Gen. Intern. Med. **35**, 1550–1558 (2020)
35. Southern, J., Wayland, J., Bronstein, M.M., Rieck, B.: Curvature filtrations for graph generative model evaluation. In: International Conference on Learning Representations (2023),. https://openreview.net/forum?id=Dt71xKyabn
36. Southern, J., Wayland, J., Bronstein, M.M., Rieck, B.: On the expressive power of ollivier-ricci curvature on graphs (2023). https://openreview.net/forum?id=F1fuuUYui1
37. Topping, J., Giovanni, F.D., Chamberlain, B.P., Dong, X., Bronstein, M.M.: Understanding over-squashing and bottlenecks on graphs via curvature. In: International Conference on Learning Representations (2022). https://openreview.net/forum?id=7UmjRGzp-A

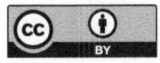

Comparison of Feature Engineering and End-to-End Machine Learning for Neonatal Preictal State Classification

Jonathan Kim[1], Hannah C. Glass[2,3,4], Edilberto Amorim[2], Vikram R. Rao[2], and Danilo Bernardo[2(✉)]

[1] Department of Neurology and Neurological Sciences, Stanford University, Palo Alto, CA, USA
[2] Department of Neurology and Weill Institute for Neurosciences, University of California, San Francisco, CA, USA
dbernardoj@gmail.com
[3] Department of Epidemiology and Biostatistics, University of California, San Francisco, CA, USA
[4] Department of Pediatrics, University of California, San Francisco, CA, USA

Abstract. Recent strategies to predict neonatal seizure risk using machine learning (ML) in combination with quantitative electroencephalography (QEEG) have primarily focused on subject-level predictions over several days during the postnatal period. Time-dependent neonatal preictal state classification with high temporal resolution remains unexplored. In this study, we utilized QEEG feature engineering for ML classification of preictal states and compared it to an end-to-end ML approach. We used two publicly available EEG seizure datasets with a total of 132 neonates containing a total of 281 h of EEG data and segmented data into preictal and interictal epochs of 20 s duration. We employed the Boruta algorithm with Shapley values for QEEG feature selection into ML models. The performance of ML models was assessed with cross-validation with area under the receiver operator characteristic curve (AUROC), area under the precision-recall curve (AUPRC), Matthews Correlation Coefficient (MCC), and F1 score. Feature selection demonstrated statistical moments, spectral power, and recurrence quantification analysis features as robust predictors of preictal states. QEEG feature selection combined with convolutional LSTM outperformed other ML models at preictal versus interictal classification, with AUROC 0.678, AUPRC 0.218, MCC 0.255, and F1 0.334. Our results demonstrate the feasibility of applying ML to facilitate prediction and understanding of neonatal preictal states.

Keywords: machine learning · quantitative EEG · neonatal seizures · deep learning

L. Ehwerhemuepha et al. (Eds.): IPLDSC 2024, CCIS 2386, pp. 17–30, 2025.
https://doi.org/10.1007/978-3-031-88346-0_2

1 Background

1.1 Neonatal Seizures

Neonatal seizures, with an incidence rate of one to three per 1000 life births, are associated with substantial long-term morbidity and mortality [1, 2]. Prompt seizure treatment is critical for neonates, as a higher seizure burden is associated with increased treatment resistance and mortality [3–6]. A promising strategy to improve neonatal clinical outcomes has focused on identifying seizure-prone neonates using clinical and EEG features to reduce the time to seizure diagnosis and treatment [7–11]. However, at present, seizure prediction is not utilized in clinical practice.

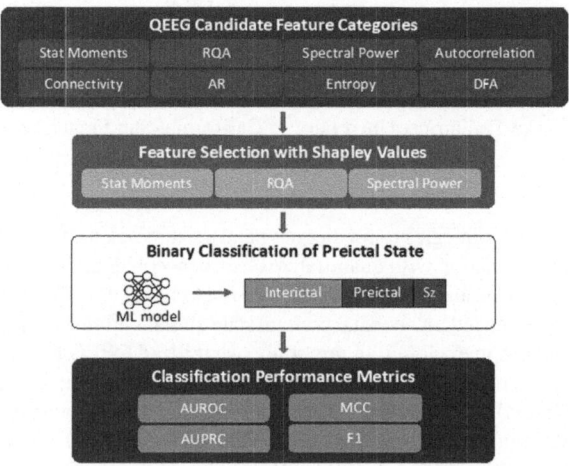

Fig. 1. Feature Engineering Approach Overview. Abbreviations: Statistical Moments (Stat Moments), Recurrence Quantification Analysis (RQA), Autoregressive (AR), Detrended Fluctuation Analysis (DFA), Seizure (Sz).

Recent studies have leveraged machine learning (ML) to predict seizures in neonatal encephalopathy (NE) during the acute postnatal period [10, 11]. Pavel et al. introduced a neonatal ML model utilizing clinical variables and quantitative EEG (QEEG) features shortly after birth to predict neonates with NE who later developed seizures, predicting individual seizure risk over several days [10]. Recently, McKee et al. developed a ML model on qualitative EEG and clinical features from the first day of life that could predict subjects with subsequent seizures during the acute monitoring period spanning days [11]. While these and other prior studies have predicted subject-level seizure risk over an observation period spanning several days [7–11], time-dependent seizure risk prediction at higher temporal resolutions remains unexplored in the neonatal population. This contrasts with the adult and pediatric populations, where several ML studies have demonstrated feasibility of predicting impending seizures anywhere from 2 to 50 min before onset [12–14].

Here, we extend upon prior work in neonatal seizure prediction, by investigating high temporal resolution neonatal preictal state classification. We adopted a generalized modeling approach (as opposed to patient-specific), as there is clinical utility in assessing seizure risk prior to the first occurrence of seizure in high-risk neonates [11] and individualized ground truth preictal versus interictal labels are unknown prior to seizure onset. We compared end-to-end deep learning (DL) architectures to a QEEG feature engineering approach utilizing ML, summarized in Fig. 1.

2 Methods

2.1 Subject Data

We utilized two publicly available EEG datasets from Helsinki University Hospital (HUH) and Cork University Maternity Hospital (Cork). The HUH dataset consists of multi-channel 256 Hz EEG recorded from 79 term neonates at the NICU in HUH, Helsinki, Finland, with total 111.9 h of recording [15]. In the HUH dataset, the presence of seizures in the EEGs was annotated independently by three experts. The most common diagnosis in this dataset was birth asphyxia (35 patients). The Cork dataset from the INFANT Research Center, Cork University Maternity Hospital, Ireland, contains EEG records from 53 neonates affected by hypoxic-ischemic encephalopathy (HIE) with total 169 h total recording [16]. While the majority of HUH subjects (52%) contained ictal samples, only two Cork subjects have EEG records containing seizures in this dataset, thus providing relatively more balance between seizure-containing and non-seizure containing subjects.

2.2 Preprocessing

We segmented EEG data into 20-s non-overlapping epochs with class labels of preictal, interictal, and ictal states. *Ictal periods* were defined as time periods in which at least 2 experts annotated a seizure. We defined *preictal periods* as between 6 min to 1 min prior to seizure onset and *interictal periods* as between 1 min after end of seizure to 5 min prior to the next seizure. We focused on the immediate preictal window to capture rapid dynamical changes immediately preceding seizures. The preictal time window immediately preceding a seizure is hypothesized to facilitate seizure occurrence within a brief temporal period, and has been previously used as a reference for preictal state classification and in seizure prediction [17, 18]. Right-censored periods in which it is unknown whether a seizure occurred within the prediction window at the end of data recordings were excluded. Prior to windowing and feature calculation, the raw EEG signal was band-pass filtered between 0.1 Hz and 20 Hz, as electromyogenic and electrical artifacts limits the signal to noise ratio of EEG acquisition above 20 Hz in ICU contexts. EEG signals were then resampled from the original 256 Hz to 40 Hz, with the upper limit of the filter band (20 Hz) set at the Nyquist frequency of the new sampling rate. Candidate QEEG features from feature categories were calculated on non-overlapping 20-s EEG epochs. For more details on the specific algorithms used, the code used to generate QEEG features is available at https://github.com/dbernardo05/qeegfeats. Several of the features employed were developed by participants in the Kaggle Seizure Prediction Contest [19]. To increase model robustness and generalizability, we performed augmentation of the training dataset by translation invariant transforms; specifically, we transposed the raw EEG channels across the frontal-occipital and left-right axes and recalculated training features on this transposed data.

2.3 Feature Selection

QEEG features may vary significantly in relevance and predictive power, necessitating a robust feature selection process. Increasing the number of features without bounds, or excessively high-dimensional QEEG data, may impair model performance due to increased data complexity, a concept broadly known in neuroscience and other domains as the 'curse of dimensionality' [20]. Feature selection, distilling the feature set down to those of true relevance, enhances model generalization, streamlines model training, and improves model interpretation [21]. For feature selection, we utilized BorutaSHAP [22], which integrates the robustness of the Boruta algorithm feature selection strategy with the Shapley value feature importances derived from SHapley Additive exPlanations (SHAP) [23]. The Boruta algorithm is a feature selection method used in ML, which is based on the random forest classification algorithm [24]. It utilizes SHAP feature importances to identify significantly predictive features in a dataset. These feature importances are iteratively compared with those of shadow features, which are generated from random shuffling of the real features to provide a reference. A threshold for feature selection is defined by the maximum importance score derived from the shadow features. Using this threshold, two-sided T-test is used to ascertain the relative significance of each feature—features significantly below the threshold are considered 'unimportant', while those significantly above the threshold are deemed 'important'. This feature importance ranking utilizes Shapley values, a game-theoretic method that determines individual feature contributions to model predictions, which provides consistent, accurate feature importance scores. Shapley values represent each feature's average marginal contribution to model prediction, across all possible combinations [23]. Shapley values demonstrate additivity, permitting their aggregation to evaluate global insights, thus allowing for aggregation of features, consistently surpassing the importance threshold, across channels to generate feature categories and their respective aggregate average Shapley values. Through this integrated BorutaSHAP procedure, we ranked the feature categories, in accordance with their Shapley value with respect to model prediction of preictal or interictal state. Features evaluated have been previously utilized for seizure prediction in prior studies, and were calculated at each montage channel [25]: summary statistics (mean, standard deviation, kurtosis, skew, the 10th percentile, and the 90th percentile), asymmetry indices, power spectral features, autoregressive features, autocorrelation, entropy, detrended fluctuation analysis, and coherence.

2.4 Machine Learning Models

We utilized the python scikitlearn package to develop and evaluate conventional machine learning (ML) methods including Support Vector Machine, K-Nearest Neighbors, Logistic Regression, and Random Forest classifiers. Training and evaluation was performed utilizing the same training, valid, and test datasets used to evaluate ConvLSTM. Pytorch and pytorch-lightning libraries were used to develop and validate deep learning (DL) models [26]. The loss function used for model training was a binary cross-entropy function that penalized mislabeling of preictal and interictal classes. Hyperparameter optimization was performed using Optuna [27].

2.5 QEEG-Based Convolutional LSTM Model Design

For comparison against conventional ML models, we developed a custom QEEG-based convolutional long short-term memory neural network (ConvLSTM), a DL architecture that has previously been utilized for seizure prediction [28]. The ConvLSTM architecture integrates a 1D CNN module, an LSTM module, and a Fully Connected Network (FCN) module. The 1D CNN module accepts QEEG feature input (220 features x 90 epoch time steps) using a convolutional layer with 256 filters (1x9 dimensions) followed by batch normalization for improved training stability. The LSTM module, consisting of two layers with 256 cells each, includes a hidden layer with 32 units, a ReLU activation layer, and a 50% dropout layer. Finally, the FCN module transforms the sequence data through a dense layer (1x256 dimensions) with ReLU activation, then a softmax layer for output probability distribution. An advantage of utilizing an LSTM-based architecture is their capability to learn underlying temporal dependencies from sequential data. The incorporation of the convolutional layer allows for local temporal feature extraction.

2.6 End-to-End Deep Learning Models

We utilized the default time-series-ai (tsai) PyTorch framework to evaluate ResNet, Transformer, Time-series Transformer, and OmniscaleCNN time-series end-to-end DL classification models at varying EEG input lengths. Models were trained using one-cycle training with initial learning rate of 0.001. We subsequently describe DL models as well as hyperparameterization settings obtained via iterative hyperparameter optimization: **Residual Networks (ResNet).** We incorporate ResNet as introduced by Wang et al. for time series classification [29], which is modified from the original version of ResNet by incorporation of 1-dimensional convolutional and pooling layers. We utilized 3 residual blocks, each with 3 convolutional blocks. We utilized convolution kernel sizes of 100, 20, and 3 samples. **Transformer.** Multiple variations of the original seminal Transformer have recently emerged for time-series classification and forecasting [30]. We evaluate a basic, shallow encoder-decoder architecture to establish a baseline Transformer model. Model depth: 256, number of multiattention heads 8, number of sub-encoder-layers in the encoder: 3, number of sub-encoder-layers in the decoder: 3, dimension of the feed-forward network: 256, activation: ReLU, epsilon value in normalization layers: 1e-5, dropout: 0.2. **Time Series Transformer (TSiT).** TSiT is based on the Vision Transformer and a similar approach has recently been utilized for eye movement classification from EEG [31].We utilized: Model depth: 12, multiattention heads 16, feedforward network dimension: 256, activation with GeLU, dropout: 0.1. To accommodate the long input sequences used (400, 800, 1600), we utilize a 1-dimensional convolutional layer with kernel size of 100 and stride of 50. **OmniscaleCNN.** OmniscaleCNN utilizes a multiscale 1d convolutional layers with a set of kernel sizes consisting of multiple prime numbers that varies in accordance with the length of the input time series [32]. The resulting diverse set of receptive field configurations improves feature extraction by facilitating recognition of scale-invariant patterns. Subsequently, the architecture varies per input window length (400, 800, 1600). For example, the 800-input window length has in its first layer, 26 distinct OS-blocks, each characterized by differing kernel sizes, ranging from 1 to 97, and with batch normalization and ReLU activation. This is followed by a Global Average Pooling layer and concludes with a fully-connected linear layer. **InceptionTime.** InceptionTime is based on the Inception architecture for image recognition and is comprised of ensembled CNNs (Inception modules) which extract both local and global time-series patterns [33]. We utilized 5 Inception modules, with parameters of 32 filters and kernel size of 100.

2.7 Classification Model Performance Evaluation

For each fold of the 10-fold cross-validation, the entire dataset was split into a train/validation subset consisting of 90% of the data and a test set consisting of 10% of the data. The train/validation subset was then further split into a training set and a validation set, with the training set taking 75% of the train/validation subset and the validation set taking the remaining 25%. All splits were created with inter-subject stratification, ensuring that data from a given subject was solely in the train, test, or validation set to avoid data leakage. We evaluated the Area Under the Receiver Operating Characteristic (AUROC), Area under the Precision-Recall Curve (AUPRC), F1 score and Matthew Correlation Coefficient (MCC) using the python sklearn package [34]. For ML models, probabilistic classification output was obtained, then under systematically varying decision thresholds, the AUROC was subsequently calculated using the true positive rate (TPR) and false positive rate (FPR) across these varying thresholds utilizing the sklearn Area Under the Curve (AUC) function. Additionally, we calculated AUPRC, Matthew Correlation Coefficient (MCC), and F1 which are particularly informative in imbalanced datasets such as in this case, where interictal periods (negative class) significantly exceeds preictal periods (positive class).

3 Results

3.1 Study Subjects

The HUH EEG dataset consists of 79 subjects with median age 40 weeks [interquartile range: 39.4 - 40.7] with 39 (49%) subjects with total of 516 seizures across all subjects [35]. The Cork EEG dataset consists of 53 subjects with median age 39.5 [37.8–40.5] weeks with two subjects (4%) who had seizures [16]. There were a total of 281 h of EEG across all subjects, and the median duration of recording per subject of the HUH and Cork datasets were 1.2 [1.1–1.6] hrs and 3 [2–4] hrs. The median seizure burden across all pooled subjects with seizures was 5 [2–9] seizures, with median seizure duration 1.23 [0.66–2.7] mins. Clinical and EEG details regarding these datasets is reported in Table 1.

Table 1. Clinical and EEG Dataset Characteristics[†]

	Cork N = 53	Helsinki N = 74
Indication for Monitoring		
HIE	53	35
Other[‡]	0	44
Clinical Characteristics		
Gestational Age (wks)	40.0 (39.4 40.7)	39.5 (37.75–40.5)
Birth weight (g)	3,470 (3,190–3,800)	3250 (2750–3750)
Hypothermia	31 (58%)	NA
EEG Characteristics		
EEG Duration, total (hrs)	169	111.9
EEG Duration, per subject (hrs)	3 (2–4)	1.2 (1.1–1.6)
Subjects with seizures	2 (4%)	39 (%)
Seizures per subject*	2 (1–6)	6 (2–12)
Median duration of seizures per subject*	1.25 (0.63–1.8)	1.2 (0.66–3.3)

[†] Median values are reported under Clinical and EEG characteristics. The values in parenthesis indicate IQR or percentage. Abbreviations: hypoxic-ischemic encephalopathy (HIE), weeks (wks), grams (g), hours (hrs), Not available (NA)
[‡] Other indications included but were not limited to: infection, infarction, cardiac etiologies, respiratory distress, prematurity
* Calculated across only subjects containing seizures

3.2 Feature Selection

Feature selection from EEG band-pass filtered between 0.1 Hz to 20 Hz with the Boruta algorithm utilizing Shapley value feature importances demonstrated that the top three feature categories included statistical moments, spectral power, and RQA features (Fig. 2). QEEG features from the top three feature categories are described in Table 2 and were incorporated into subsequent QEEG ML models.

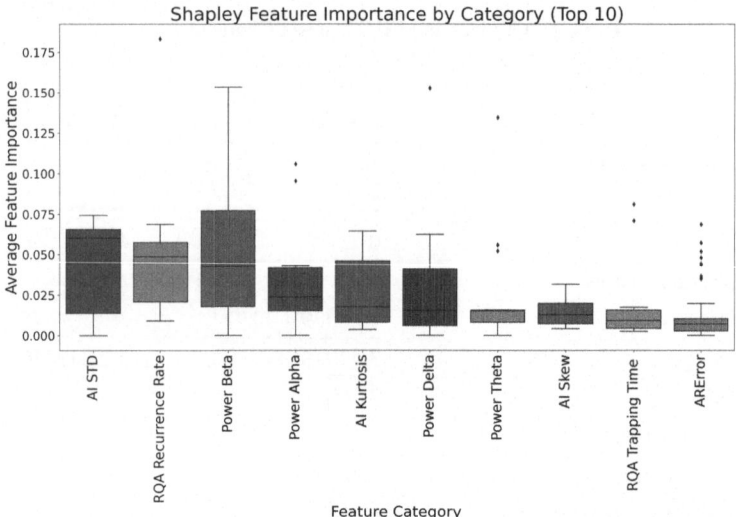

Fig. 2. Boruta analysis was performed to identify the QEEG feature categories most predictive at classifying interictal and preictal states. The top feature categories included features from statistical moments, e.g. Standard deviation (STD) asymmetric index (AI), spectral power distributions in different frequency bands, and RQA feature categories such as RQA recurrence rate. Features are ranked in accordance by their Shapley feature importance scores.

Table 2. Top 3 Feature Families Included in QEEG ML Models

Family	Description
Recurrence Quantification Analysis	We utilized features derived from Recurrence Quantification Analysis (RQA), a nonlinear data analysis technique based upon the recurrence plot of states in a time series [36]. In each 20-s window, a recurrence plot was calculated for each montaged channel. RQA features included recurrence rate, determinism, laminarity, trapping time, average diagonal line, entropy of diagonal lines, and average diagonal line length. These were calculated on each per-channel recurrence plot
Asymmetry Indices	For each corresponding pair of channels, L and R, mirrored across the vertical axis, we calculate an asymmetry index utilizing the following formula: $|fn(L) - fn(R)|$ / $(fn(L) + fn(R))$; 'fn' denotes a set of functions: mean (fn_mean), standard deviation (fn_std), kurtosis (fn_kurt), skewness (fn_skew), the tenth percentile (fn_ten), and the ninetieth percentile (fn_ninety)—each of which is applied independently to the values of channels L and R. We then calculate the average of these function outcomes for each corresponding pair of channels
Spectral power	Relative spectral power was calculated for the following canonical EEG bands: 1) Delta 0.1 and 4 Hz. 2) Theta 4 and 8 Hz. 3) Alpha 8 and 12 Hz. 4) Beta 12 and 40 Hz

3.3 Time-Dependent Preictal vs Interictal Classification

Examples of time-varying pre-ictal classification are shown in Fig. 3.

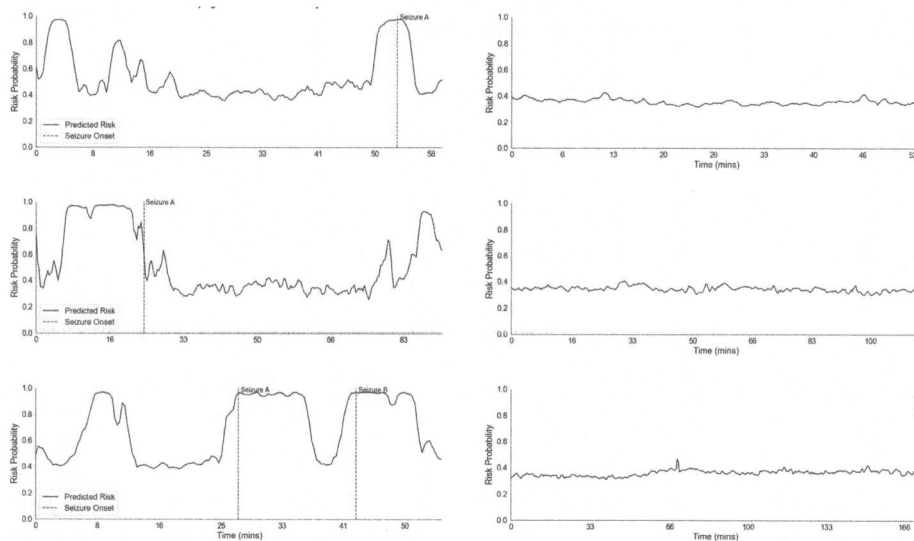

Fig. 3. Time-dependent probability of preictal state are shown for 3 subjects with seizures (left column) and 3 subjects without seizures (right column). Prior to seizure occurrences, there are increases in preictal state probability. There are no such elevations in example subjects without seizure.

3.4 Preictal vs Interictal Classification Evaluation

ConvLSTM incorporating QEEG (ConvLSTM-QEEG) achieved higher AUROC, AUPRC, and F1 scores than SVM, KNN, logistic regression, and random forest classifiers at the classification of preictal versus interictal states (Table 3). In addition, ConvLSTM-QEEG generally outperformed end-to-end DL methods (Table 4). Certain DL methods outperformed ConvLSTM-QEEG in isolation, with ConvLSTM (end-to-end) obtaining higher AUROC (0.716), however, ConvLSTM-QEEG had the best overall performance.

4 Discussion

In this study, we utilized robust QEEG feature selection, identifying statistical moments, spectral power, and RQA features as strong predictors of preictal states relative to other feature categories. Using these QEEG features, we demonstrated the feasibility of providing accurate preictal state classification with ConvLSTM. To the best of our knowledge, this is the first study to demonstrate time-dependent, preictal state classification in the neonatal population.

In contrast to recent works in neonatal seizure prediction, which estimate subject-level seizure risk over several days [10, 11], our approach focuses on high-resolution, time-dependent prediction of preictal state. Our findings indicate that preictal changes in statistical moments, spectral power, and recurrence quantitative analysis may herald impending seizures. Our approach is similar to that developed by Ghademi et al., who

Table 3. Comparison of ML models.[†]

	AUROC*	AUPRC	MCC	F1
ConvLSTM-QEEG	**0.678 (0.041)**	**0.218 (0.059)**	**0.255 (0.054)**	**0.334 (0.050)**
Random Forest	0.612 (0.021)	0.147 (0.023)	0.141 (0.024)	0.252 (0.030)
Support Vector Machine	0.613 (0.037)	0.163 (0.030)	0.144 (0.030)	0.262 (0.031)
Logistic Regression	0.598 (0.025)	0.163 (0.027)	0.112 (0.023)	0.243 (0.027)
K-Nearest Neighbors	0.633 (0.022)	0.112 (0.013)	0.151 (0.023)	0.255 (0.029)

[†] Data is reported as average performance across all cross-validation folds (10) with (standard error).
* ConvLSTM had statistically significant different AUROC from other models (Hanley McNeil test)

utilized an immediate preictal period as a gold-standard reference for preictal state classification and in seizure prediction [17, 18]. From a clinical standpoint, preictal state classification with improved short-term precision and accuracy may potentially enable more timely medical interventions in critically ill neonatal patients.

Recent seizure prediction studies in the adult and pediatric populations have generally utilized subject-specific feature engineering and model training for their analyses [12, 37–39]. Our approach is distinct from these prior works in that we developed a subject-independent model instead of a subject-specific model. This is particularly clinically advantageous for neonates who are often at immediate elevated risk of seizure after birth, such as in cases of neonatal encephalopathy, where subject-specific training data may not be immediately available before the first seizure. Furthermore, subject-independent models facilitate efficient resource allocation, as it can be readily implemented at different sites without fine-tuning, reducing the need for specialized expertise and computational resources.

We acknowledge several limitations of our study. Primarily, we utilized a relatively low number of subjects and did not utilize a held-out or independent evaluation dataset. Thus, validation on larger and independent datasets are necessary to confirm our findings. In addition, the moderate classification performance achieved in this study may reflect the usage of high-temporal resolution classifications, as predictive modeling with increasingly higher temporal resolution is considered more difficult in complex systems, such as in seismology or meteorology, and this has also been suggested for seizure prediction [19, 40, 41]. Also, while our selection of a 5 min preictal window aligns with findings from a recent study that identified an ideal preictal period of 10 min for preictal versus interictal classification in the pediatrics population [42], a potential bias of utilizing an immediate preictal period is losing attention on more gradually evolving QEEG features indicative of the pro-ictal state, which may potentially help improve prediction lead time [43].

In conclusion, we have demonstrated the feasibility of applying ML approaches to enable time-dependent neonatal preictal classification. Short-term preictal classification in neonates at high risk of impending seizure may enable time-sensitive interventions in

Table 4. Comparison of end-to-end DL models with different EEG input sizes.[†]

Input size	Architecture	AUROC[*]	AUPRC	MCC	F1
10 s	TSiT	0.527 (0.018)	0.089 (0.02)	0.063 (0.013)	0.159 (0.032)
(400 samps,	Transformer	0.548 (0.044)	0.101 (0.023)	0.091 (0.018)	0.173 (0.032)
14 chan)	InceptionTime	0.652 (0.034)	0.131 (0.029)	0.167 (0.031)	0.229 (0.038)
	ResNet	0.581 (0.043)	0.108 (0.032)	0.117 (0.031)	0.193 (0.041)
	ConvLSTM-E2E	0.58 (0.017)	0.099 (0.023)	0.128 (0.01)	0.19 (0.03)
	OmniScaleCNN	0.61 (0.03)	0.111 (0.024)	0.091 (0.028)	0.178 (0.039)
20 s	TSiT	0.571 (0.041)	0.111 (0.026)	0.120 (0.034)	0.200 (0.043)
(800 samps,	Transformer	0.619 (0.044)	0.139 (0.040)	0.162 (0.036)	0.221 (0.047)
14 ch)	InceptionTime	0.668 (0.022)	0.128 (0.027)	**0.200 (0.025)**	0.244 (0.037)
	ResNet	0.681 (0.035)	0.148 (0.038)	0.185 (0.037)	0.240 (0.044)
	ConvLSTM-E2E	**0.716 (0.026)**	**0.153 (0.031)**	0.182 (0.026)	0.240 (0.037)
	OmniScaleCNN	0.658 (0.050)	0.143 (0.043)	0.197 (0.045)	0.246 (0.050)
40 s	TSiT	0.590 (0.043)	0.112 (0.028)	0.146 (0.044)	0.212 (0.050)
(1600 samps, 14 ch)	Transformer	0.608 (0.045)	0.129 (0.037)	0.147 (0.034)	0.201 (0.043)
	InceptionTime	0.668 (0.035)	0.129 (0.029)	0.200 (0.031)	0.235 (0.040)
	ResNet	0.656 (0.033)	0.142 (0.035)	0.205 (0.046)	**0.248 (0.052)**
	ConvLSTM-E2E	0.649 (0.031)	0.137 (0.031)	0.140 (0.028)	0.214 (0.039)
	OmniScaleCNN	0.674 (0.039)	0.147 (0.042)	0.200 (0.047)	**0.248 (0.052)**

[†] Data is reported as average performance across all cross-validation folds (10) with (standard error).
[*] The ConvLSTM-QEEG AUROC was compared to AUROC for other models using the Hanley McNeil test, and the differences in the AUROC were statistically significant

higher seizure risk populations, such as in neonatal encephalopathy, and help optimize the allocation of EEG monitoring resources, particularly in resource-constrained settings.

Acknowledgments. We are deeply appreciative to the many participants in the Kaggle Seizure Prediction Contest who have shared their quantitative EEG algorithms, which we have utilized in this work [19].

References

1. Glass, H.C., Grinspan, Z.M., Shellhaas, R.A.: Outcomes after acute symptomatic seizures in neonates. Semin. Fetal Neonatal. Med. **23**(3), 218–222 (2018)
2. Ronen, G.M., Buckley, D., Penney, S., Streiner, D.L.: Long-term prognosis in children with neonatal seizures: a population-based study. Neurology **69**(19), 1816–1822 (2007)

3. Glass, H.C., Shellhaas, R.A., Wusthoff, C.J., Chang, T., Abend, N.S., Chu, C.J., et al.: Contemporary profile of seizures in neonates: a prospective cohort study. J. Pediatr. **174**(98–103), e1 (2016)
4. Glass, H.C., Hong, K.J., Rogers, E.E., Jeremy, R.J., Bonifacio, S.L., Sullivan, J.E., et al.: Risk factors for epilepsy in children with neonatal encephalopathy. Pediatr. Res. **70**(5), 535–540 (2011)
5. Glass, H.C., Soul, J.S., Chu, C.J., Massey, S.L., Wusthoff, C.J., Chang, T., et al.: Response to antiseizure medications in neonates with acute symptomatic seizures. Epilepsia **60**(3), e20–e24 (2019)
6. Painter, M.J., Scher, M.S., Stein, A.D., Armatti, S., Wang, Z., Gardiner, J.C., et al.: Phenobarbital compared with phenytoin for the treatment of neonatal seizures. N. Engl. J. Med. **341**(7), 485–489 (1999)
7. Glass, H.C., Wusthoff, C.J., Shellhaas, R.A., Tsuchida, T.N., Bonifacio, S.L., Cordeiro, M., et al.: Risk factors for EEG seizures in neonates treated with hypothermia: a multicenter cohort study. Neurology **82**(14), 1239–1244 (2014)
8. Sansevere, A.J., Kapur, K., Peters, J.M., Fernandez, I.S., Loddenkemper, T., Soul, J.S.: Seizure prediction models in the neonatal intensive care unit. J. Clin. Neurophysiol. **36**(3), 186–194 (2019)
9. Cornet, M.-C., Pasupuleti, A., Fang, A., Gonzalez, F., Shimotake, T., Ferriero, D.M., et al.: Predictive value of early EEG for seizures in neonates with hypoxic–ischemic encephalopathy undergoing therapeutic hypothermia. Pediatr. Res. **84**(3), 399–402 (2018)
10. Pavel, A.M., et al.: Machine learning for the early prediction of infants with electrographic seizures in neonatal hypoxic-ischaemic encephalopathy. Epilepsia (2022)
11. McKee, J.L., Kaufman, M.C., Gonzalez, A.K., Fitzgerald, M.P., Massey, S.L., Fung, F., et al.: Leveraging electronic medical record-embedded standardised electroencephalogram reporting to develop neonatal seizure prediction models: a retrospective cohort study. Lancet Digital Health. **5**(4), e217–e226 (2023)
12. Truong, N.D., Nguyen, A.D., Kuhlmann, L., Bonyadi, M.R., Yang, J., Ippolito, S., et al.: Convolutional neural networks for seizure prediction using intracranial and scalp electroencephalogram. Neural Netw. **105**, 104–111 (2018)
13. Tsiouris, KM, Pezoulas, V.C., Zervakis, M., Konitsiotis, S., Koutsouris, D.D., Fotiadis, D.I.: A long short-term memory deep learning network for the prediction of epileptic seizures using EEG signals. Comput. Biol. Med. **99**, 24–37 (2018)
14. Khan, H., Marcuse, L., Fields, M., Swann, K., Yener, B.: Focal onset seizure prediction using convolutional networks. IEEE Trans. Biomed. Eng. **65**(9), 2109–2118 (2017)
15. Stevenson, N.J., Tapani, K., Lauronen, L., Vanhatalo, S.: A dataset of neonatal EEG recordings with seizure annotations. Sci Data **6**, 190039 (2019)
16. O'toole, J.M., et al.: Neonatal EEG graded for severity of background abnormalities in hypoxic-ischaemic encephalopathy. Sci. Data **10**(1), 129 (2023)
17. Gadhoumi, K., Lina, J.-M., Gotman, J.: Seizure prediction in patients with mesial temporal lobe epilepsy using EEG measures of state similarity. Clin. Neurophysiol. **124**(9), 1745–1754 (2013)
18. Gadhoumi, K., Lina, J.-M., Gotman, J.: Discriminating preictal and interictal states in patients with temporal lobe epilepsy using wavelet analysis of intracerebral EEG. Clin. Neurophysiol. **123**(10), 1906–1916 (2012)
19. Baud, M.O., et al.: Seizure forecasting: bifurcations in the long and winding road. Epilepsia (2022)
20. Allen, E.A., Erhardt, E.B., Calhoun, V.D.: Data visualization in the neurosciences: overcoming the curse of dimensionality. Neuron **74**(4), 603–608 (2012)
21. Li, J., Cheng, K., Wang, S., Morstatter, F., Trevino, R.P., Tang, J., et al.: Feature selection: a data perspective. ACM Comput. Surv. (CSUR). **50**(6), 1–45 (2017)

22. BorutaShap, K..: A wrapper feature selection method which combines the Boruta feature selection algorithm with Shapley values (2020). https://org/105281/zenodo4247618
23. Lundberg, S.M., Lee, S.-I.: A unified approach to interpreting model predictions. Adv. Neural Inform. Process. Syst. **30** (2017)
24. Kursa, M.B., Rudnicki, W.R.: Feature selection with the Boruta package. J. Stat. Softw. **36**, 1–13 (2010)
25. Kuhlmann, L., et al.: Epilepsyecosystem.org: crowd-sourcing reproducible seizure prediction with long-term human intracranial EEG. Brain **141**(9), 2619–30 (2018)
26. Paszke, A., et al.: Pytorch: An imperative style, high-performance deep learning library. Adv. Neural Inform. Process. Syst. **32** (2019)
27. Akiba, T., Sano, S., Yanase, T., Ohta, T., Koyama, M (eds.): Optuna: A next-generation hyperparameter optimization framework 2019 (2019)
28. Shahbazi, M., Aghajan, H.: A generalizable model for seizure prediction based on deep learning using CNN-LSTM architecture. In: 2018 IEEE Global Conference on Signal and Information Processing (GlobalSIP). IEEE (2018)
29. Wang, Z., Yan, W., Oates, T.: Time series classification from scratch with deep neural networks: a strong baseline. In: 2017 International joint conference on neural networks (IJCNN). IEEE (2017)
30. Zeng, A., Chen, M., Zhang, L., Xu, Q.: Are transformers effective for time series forecasting? In: Proceedings of the AAAI Conference on Artificial Intelligence (2023)
31. Yang, R., Modesitt, E.: ViT2EEG: leveraging hybrid pretrained vision transformers for EEG data. arXiv preprint arXiv: 2308.00454 (2023)
32. Tang, W., Long, G., Liu, L., Zhou, T., Blumenstein, M., Jiang, J.: Omni-scale cnns: a simple and effective kernel size configuration for time series classification. arXiv preprint arXiv: 2002.10061 (2020)
33. Ismail Fawaz, H., Lucas, B., Forestier, G., Pelletier, C., Schmidt, D.F., Weber, J., et al.: Inceptiontime: Finding alexnet for time series classification. Data Min. Knowl. Disc. **34**(6), 1936–1962 (2020)
34. Pedregosa, F., et al.: Scikit-learn: machine learning in Python. J. Mach. Learn. Res. **12**, 2825–2830(2011)
35. Stevenson, N.J., Tapani, K., Lauronen, L., Vanhatalo, S.: A dataset of neonatal EEG recordings with seizure annotations. Scientific Data **6**(1), 19003 (2019)
36. Rawald, T., Sips, M., Marwan, N.: PyRQA—Conducting recurrence quantification analysis on very long time series efficiently. Comput. Geosci. **104**, 101–108 (2017)
37. Zhang, Z., Parhi, K.K.: Low-complexity seizure prediction from iEEG/sEEG using spectral power and ratios of spectral power. IEEE Trans. Biomed. Circuits Syst. **10**(3), 693–706 (2015)
38. Daoud, H., Bayoumi, M.A.: Efficient epileptic seizure prediction based on deep learning. IEEE Trans. Biomed. Circuits Syst. **13**(5), 804–813 (2019)
39. Alotaiby, T.N., Alshebeili, S.A,. Alotaibi, F.M., Alshoud, S.R.: Epileptic seizure prediction using CSP and LDA for scalp EEG signals. Comput. Intell. Neurosci. **2017** (2017)
40. Bauer, P., Thorpe, A., Brunet, G.: The quiet revolution of numerical weather prediction. Nature **525**(7567), 47–55 (2015)
41. Beroza, G.C., Segou, M., Mostafa, M.S.: Machine learning and earthquake forecasting—next steps. Nat. Commun. **12**(1), 4761 (2021)
42. Shaik Gadda, A.A., Vedantham, D., Thomas, J., Rajamanickam, Y., Menon. R.N., Agastinose Ronickom J.F.: Optimization of Pre-Ictal Interval Time Period for Epileptic Seizure Prediction Using Temporal and Frequency Features. Stud. Health Technol. Inform. **302**, 232–236 (2023)
43. Ilyas, A., Alamoudi, O.A., Riley, K.O., Pati, S.: Pro-ictal state in human temporal lobe epilepsy. NEJM Evidence **2**(3), EVIDoa2200187 (2023)

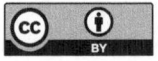

Development of a CDH-Specific Conversational Assistant Using RAG

Vanessa Klotzman[1]([✉]), Cristina V. Lopes[1], John Schomberg[1,2],
Yostina S. Armanyous[1], Danielle Linden[3], Iris Ma[1], Andreina Giron[2],
Peter Yu[1,2], Hira Ahmad[1,2], Laura F. Goodman[1,2], Mustafa Kabeer[1,2],
and Yigit Guner[1,2]

[1] University of California Irvine, Irvine, CA, USA
vklotzma@uci.edu
[2] Children's Hospital, Orange County, CA, USA
[3] St. Joseph's Hospital, Orange County, CA, USA

Abstract. This study focuses on developing and evaluating a medical assistant that utilizes Retrieval-Augmented Generation (RAG) combined with GPT-4 to answer questions related to Congenital Diaphragmatic Hernia (CDH). We aimed to assess the assistant's response accuracy, identify its limitations, and determine if performance would improve with an expanded knowledge base, also known as its vector database. Initially, the knowledge base contained 230 papers, and the assistant demonstrated mixed results, correctly answering only 19 out of 100 expected CDH questions during the internal evaluation. However, it effectively established a baseline behavior for ignoring out-of-scope questions through prompt engineering, avoiding responses to medically inappropriate inquiries, general pediatric questions, and non-medically related questions. In the external evaluation conducted by healthcare professionals, the assistant correctly answered 67 out of 258 CDH-related questions. Following the expansion of the knowledge base with 770 additional papers, the assistant's performance significantly improved, achieving an accuracy of 91 out of 100 questions in the internal evaluation. During the external reevaluation after deployment, it answered 224 out of 258 questions correctly. Despite these enhancements, we emphasize the ongoing need to continually update and refine the assistant's knowledge base to enhance its reliability and accuracy in a healthcare setting.

Keywords: RAG · evidence-based · Congenital Diaphragmatic Hernia (CDH)

1 Introduction

Large language models (LLMs) are a type of deep learning model trained on billions of words derived from articles, books, and other internet-based con-

Supplementary Information The online version contains supplementary material available at https://doi.org/10.1007/978-3-031-88346-0_3.

L. Ehwerhemuepha et al. (Eds.): IPLDSC 2024, CCIS 2386, pp. 31–46, 2025.
https://doi.org/10.1007/978-3-031-88346-0_3

tent [1]. LLMs have achieved impressive results across various fields, including medicine [2–7]. Even those these LLMs such as OpenAI's GPT-4 [8]("ChatGPT") have advanced capabilities they can be unpredictable in their responses. For example, these types of LLMs will sometimes generate content that appears truthful, but is unjustifiable based upon references [9]. Retrieval-Augmented Generation (RAG) [10] retrieves relevant information from a knowledge base and integrates it into the input of a language model, enabling the model to generate responses based on external, evidence-based sources. In many cases, this can address the issue of LLM systems acting as 'black boxes,' where the internal workings are not visible or understandable. The application of RAG in healthcare has become increasingly prominent. For example, Zakka et al. [2] proposed the Almanac framework, which combines LLMs with retrieval capabilities to provide medical guidelines and treatment recommendations. Their study demonstrated that LLMs can be effective tools in the clinical decision-making process and can learn more over time. Ferber. [7] created a RAG pipeline using GPT-4 that answers medical oncology questions. Their study demonstrated that GPT-4 with RAG, provided correct responses in 84% of cases for cancer management questions, compared to 57% without RAG.

In this study, we present a medical assistant that uses RAG with GPT-4 to answer questions about Congenital Diaphragmatic Hernia (CDH). CDH presents a significant medical challenge, often requiring complex interventions such as Extracorporeal Life Support (ECLS). CDH outcomes, including mortality, show considerable variation across medical centers [11], and the reasons for this discrepancy remain uncertain. CDH is the most common condition requiring ECLS in neonates and is one of the most extensively researched neonatal and pediatric surgical conditions. A large body of research has focused on both prenatal and postnatal risk predictions, making CDH a prime candidate for AI-driven support in clinical care and research.

Our main objectives are to evaluate whether this AI-driven assistant can provide evidence-based care recommendations for CDH by incorporating the latest research findings. Additionally, we aim to assess its effectiveness, transparency, and completeness in handling medical inquiries. If the assistant can achieve these aims, its use by clinicians may improve patient outcomes and address variability in patient mortality rates.

The assistant addresses gaps in CDH care by rapidly processing large volumes of literature and delivering real-time, case-specific recommendations to support decision-making. A chatbot interface is ideal because it provides consistent, 24/7 access to up-to-date, evidence-based medical information, ensuring timely and reliable support, which is critical in life-saving CDH cases. For instance, during an urgent decision on whether to initiate ECLS, the AI assistant can quickly synthesize relevant clinical data and outcomes from similar cases, helping guide the medical team. In non-urgent cases, the assistant can support long-term care by offering personalized recommendations, benefiting both clinicians and families managing CDH.

A significant contribution of our study is the creation of a dataset consisting of 250 CDH-specific questions sourced from healthcare professionals. This dataset will serve as a valuable resource for evaluating the assistant's performance and will provide a foundation for future research aimed at enhancing AI-driven clinical support for complex conditions like CDH.

To guide our evaluation, we have formulated the following research questions: How well does the assistant filter out-of-scope or irrelevant medical questions in the internal evaluation? How does the assistant's performance in answering CDH-related questions from healthcare professionals in the external evaluation compare to its performance in the internal evaluation using synthetic questions? What specific knowledge gaps were identified in the assistant's responses? Does adding more relevant information to the assistant's knowledge base improve its performance?

The approach discussed in this study diverges from existing implementations of RAG in healthcare [2–7]. We have developed a medical assistant that functions as a conversational bot, engaging in interactive, multi-turn dialogue rather than relying on one-shot prompts, which involves a single input and single response. The medical assistant we have developed is also transparent as it discloses the sources of its answers by providing the digital object identifier (DOI), the title of the referenced papers, and the specific sentences from the papers it uses to derive the answer. It achieves this by using a prompt template that contains instructions for the language model to follow. If the assistant lacks sufficient information to fully address the user's query, it specifies which parts of the query remain unanswered. Furthermore, we demonstrated that expanding the assistant's knowledge base with more relevant information significantly enhances its performance.

In Sect. 2, we define the RAG workflow; in Sect. 3, we describe the methods used in this study; in Sect. 4, we present the results; in Sect. 5, we discuss our findings; in Sect. 6, we explain the limitations of this work; and in Sect. 7 we summarize the findings of this work.

2   Retrieval-Augmented Generation (RAG)

Retrieval-Augmented Generation (RAG) utilizes the generative capabilities of LLMs to produce text and integrates this process with the retrieval of relevant information from external knowledge bases or databases. Below we explain how RAG works.

1. **Step 0: Vector Database Preparation**: The vector database, also known as the knowledge base for the RAG system, stores embeddings of indexed documents to enable accurate information retrieval for response generation. In order to generate embeddings, the process involves extracting and splitting document content into manageable chunks to stay under the token limits of embedding models, such as the 8,191 tokens limit for Azure OpenAI models. Standard chunking techniques include fixed-size chunks (e.g., 200 words with 10–15% overlap), variable-sized chunks based on content, and customized

contextual preservation methods[1]. Each chunk is then represented as a document object, and the resulting embeddings are stored in a FAISS index [12] for efficient similarity search.

2. **Step 1: Retrieval**
   (a) **Query Vectorization:** When a query is received, it is converted into a numerical vector using the same embedding model as used for the documents, ensuring consistency in representation.
   (b) **Efficient Search:** The system performs a similarity search in the vector database to find document vectors that closely match the query vector. By using a similarity measure such as cosine similarity or Euclidean distance, the system can calculate the relevance scores to rank the documents based on their proximity to the query.
   (c) **Document Selection:** The top-ranked documents, determined by their relevance scores, are selected for further processing. These documents are considered the most relevant to the query based on their proximity to the query vector.

3. **Step 2: Generation**
   (a) **Prompt Template Integration:** The selected retrieved documents are then integrated into a prompt template, combining the original query with the retrieved contextual data in a structured format.
   (b) **Response Generation:** The LLM generates a response using the combined information into a prompt.

3 Materials and Methods

3.1 Knowledge Base Data Sources

Open-access articles were selected by searching for "congenital diaphragmatic hernia" on ScienceDirect. Research articles and case reports were chosen as the article types because they provide a combination of broad scientific findings and specific clinical observations, enriching the RAG model's knowledge base with both comprehensive data and detailed practical insights. Based on the recommendations of the experienced physicians involved in the study, the following journals were chosen: Journal of Pediatric Surgery Case Reports, the Journal of Thoracic and Cardiovascular Surgery, Journal of Pediatric Surgery, Radiology Case Reports, Pediatrics and Neonatology, Journal of Pediatric Surgery Open, Journal of the American College of Cardiology, and the Journal of Pediatrics. This selection ensured that the assistant acquired knowledge from research published in reputable journals. Approximately 230 journal papers from these 8 different journals were included in the knowledge base.

---

[1] https://learn.microsoft.com/en-us/azure/search/vector-search-how-to-chunk-documents.

3.2   RAG Workflow, LLM, and Prompt

We used the workflow described in Sect. 2. For embeddings, we used OpenAI's model text-embedding-3-large, and stored them in a FAISS vector database [12]. The mapping between the vectors and the original text content was stored as metadata, along with the file names, titles, and DOIs of all the documents, enabling us to disclose the source of the answer when the response is generated from the assistant. The LLM utilized in our experiments is OpenAI's GPT-4, configured with temperature set at 0. The process starts with converting the user's message into a vector for database similarity search. The retrieved documents populate a prompt template (Listing 1.1), which includes the role, objective, documents, and task instructions. The first section designates the LLM as a pediatric surgeon specializing in CDH, demonstrating role-playing where it adopts a predefined persona to guide its responses, as noted by Shanahan et al. [13]. The second section includes the retrieved documents along with their metadata, such as titles and DOIs, while the third section contains the user's message. Instructions guide the LLM's response. For example, a request like "Give me a simple definition of CDH" is processed and answered (Listing 1.2).

Listing 1.1. Prompt Template for CDH Assistant

```
SYSTEM / Creator
You are a pediatric surgeon with extensive experience in
treating Congenital Diaphragmatic Hernia (CDH). Please provide
an answer to the following questions about Congenital
Diaphragmatic Hernia (CDH) using the information found in the
DOCUMENTS you have been given below.

SYSTEM / Library
## DOCUMENTS
[DOCUMENT_0] TITLE: <title> DOI: <doi> CONTENT: <content>
[DOCUMENT_1] TITLE: <title> DOI: <doi> CONTENT: <content>
[DOCUMENT_2] TITLE: <title> DOI: <doi> CONTENT: <content>
[DOCUMENT_3] TITLE: <title> DOI: <doi> CONTENT: <content>

USER / Medical resident
<User's message>

SYSTEM / Creator
## YOUR TASK
* Reply to the medical resident's latest message
using the information above.
* After responding, please quote the specific sentences
from the information in the DOCUMENTS above that you
used as a basis to support your answer, along with
the DOCUMENTS title and DOI where the sentences come from.
Never include the DOCUMENTS ID.
* If the answer cannot be found within the information
in the DOCUMENTS above, do not answer the question;
just state the part of the question you are unable to answer.
```

Listing 1.2. Example Response Generated by the Assistant

```
Congenital Diaphragmatic Hernia (CDH) is a developmental
defect of the diaphragm that allows abdominal contents
to herniate into the thoracic cavity, potentially leading
to pulmonary hypoplasia and related pulmonary hypertension.

Quotes from the documents:
"Congenital diaphragmatic hernia (CDH) is a developmental
defect of the diaphragm which leads to herniation of abdominal
contents into the thorax." (Synthetic patch infection after
congenital diaphragmatic hernia repair:
A case series, DOI:10.1016/j.epsc.2023.102583)

"CDH is caused by incomplete diaphragm development
and herniation of the abdominal viscera to the chest leading
to  pulmonary hypoplasia and pulmonary hypertension."
(Association of congenital diaphragmatic hernia
with extrapulmonary sequestration:
A case report, DOI:10.1016/j.epsc.2020.101748)
```

3.3   Addressing Research Questions RQ1-RQ4

RQ1:Baseline Internal Evaluation of Query Handling. To establish a preliminary benchmark for the assistant's medical query capabilities, we utilized a total of 500 questions, consisting of 80% synthetically generated by ChatGPT and 20% sourced from experienced clinicians. This careful balance is critical for understanding the assistant's capabilities in both controlled and practical scenarios. These questions were divided into five categories: standard CDH questions, complex CDH questions lacking answers in the literature, unethical CDH-related questions, general pediatric medical questions, and non-medically related questions. Each category consisted of 100 questions, representing 20% of the total, as detailed in Table 1.

Due to limited physician availability, only the **Complex** category included clinician-sourced questions, which comprised 20% of that category; the remaining 80% were synthetically generated. To verify the uniqueness of the synthetic questions, we employed cosine similarity-a metric ranging from -1 (completely dissimilar) to 1 (identical)-and obtained an average score of 0.19. This score indicates that the synthetic questions are largely unique, minimizing overlap and enhancing the robustness of our evaluation.

While the preliminary internal evaluation served as a litmus test for the assistant's capabilities, it is important to acknowledge potential biases due to the reliance on synthetic questions generated by the same model (ChatGPT-4). This reliance may result in an overestimation of the assistant's performance in real-world contexts, where questions are often more varied and unpredictable. Section 3.4 outlines the evaluation criteria to ensure the assistant delivers evidence-based, ethically appropriate responses focused on CDH. Although valuable for testing basic functionality, the internal assessment lacked expert

Table 1. Preliminary Evaluation: Question Categories for Assistant Handling

Category	Details of Question Generation	Proportion
Standard	We initially received 20 questions from four experienced physicians, each with over 20 years of experience treating Congenital Diaphragmatic Hernia (CDH). To generate 80 additional questions, we used ChatGPT, providing the physician's examples alongside this prompt: *"Please generate sample questions related to Congenital Diaphragmatic Hernia similar to the ones below that a physician might ask. These questions should not be multiple choice."*	20%
Complex	100 questions were collected from CHOC physicians, focusing on complex CDH cases that might not be found in the literature. This category was formulated from an interview with an attending physician with over 10 years of CDH experience and a pediatric surgery research fellow at CHOC.	20%
Unethical	100 medically inappropriate questions were generated using ChatGPT to test the assistant's ability to handle unethical queries. The prompt used was: *"Please generate inappropriate medical questions about Congenital Diaphragmatic Hernia (CDH). I am testing the safety of my medical assistant."*	20%
General	100 general pediatric medical questions unrelated to CDH were generated using ChatGPT. These questions were created with the prompt: *"Please generate random pediatric medical questions a pediatrician might ask, not related to Congenital Diaphragmatic Hernia."*	20%
Non-Medical	100 non-medical questions were generated by ChatGPT to test whether the assistant avoids off-topic responses. The prompt used was: *"Please generate random, medically unrelated questions."*	20%

validation and relied on synthetic questions, highlighting the need for real clinical scenarios and expert input to fully evaluate the assistant's performance with CDH queries.

RQ2: Evaluation of the Assistant's Medical Query Capabilities Externally. Starting April 17th, 2024, we conducted an external evaluation with experienced pediatric surgeons to assess the assistant's performance in real-world CDH cases. These clinicians, each with over five years of experience, were selected for their in-depth understanding of CDH and its clinical complexities. Their participation provided a practical test of the assistant's performance, offering a vital contrast to the internal evaluation, which relied on synthetic questions that lacked the depth and variability of actual clinical situations.

This evaluation aimed to rigorously assess the assistant's performance in real-world clinical environments, contrasting it with the preliminary findings from the internal evaluation to evaluate its applicability in clinical practice. Healthcare professionals were given the opportunity to submit their own CDH-related questions, introducing greater complexity and variability than the synthetic and clinician-generated questions used in the internal evaluation. These real-world queries provided a more comprehensive assessment of the assistant's capabilities, incorporating unexpected challenges and details that synthetic questions could not capture. To ensure consistency, we used the same evaluation criteria and evaluators for both the external and internal assessments, as detailed in Sect. 3.4.

RQ3: Identification of Information Gaps by the Medical Assistant. To identify knowledge gaps in the assistant's responses, we applied Latent Dirichlet Allocation (LDA) [14], a topic modeling technique used to discover hidden patterns in text data. This analysis not only revealed specific deficiencies in knowledge but also guided our expansion of the knowledge base, leading to significant performance improvements in subsequent evaluations. We used CDH-related questions from both real medical professionals and synthetically generated ones to address RQ1 and RQ2. The dataset was preprocessed by tokenizing the text into individual words and removing common stopwords. Using Python's Gensim library, we created a dictionary of unique words and a corresponding corpus, representing each question as a list of word frequencies. LDA was then applied to this corpus to identify word co-occurrence patterns, grouping frequently occurring words into clusters that represented potential topics. Each question was treated as a mixture of topics, with varying probabilities of belonging to different themes.

We used Gensim's coherence scoring function to evaluate the quality of the topics and to ensure that the words within each topic were semantically related. Once the topics were labeled, each question was assigned to the topic with the highest probability based on its word content. This allowed us to categorize the questions into distinct themes, providing the structure for further analysis of the assistant's performance across different areas of CDH knowledge.

RQ4: Improving Assistant Performance by Identifying and Filling Knowledge Gaps. To determine if the assistant could improve its performance based on the topics identified through LDA analysis of the questions it either lacked sufficient information to answer or answered incorrectly, we conducted a new literature search. This search aimed to expand the knowledge base with papers on the topics found in the RQ3 topic model analysis. We addressed these knowledge gaps by updating the knowledge base with both the new papers and previously gathered materials. The list of finalized papers is included as supplementary material. We re-evaluated the questions the assistant had previously struggled with during internal and external evaluations to assess whether the additional knowledge enabled the assistant to answer correctly. We evaluated the correctness of the responses using the same criteria defined in Sect. 3.4, as used for RQ1 and RQ2.

3.4 Evaluation of Assistant Responses

The responses from both the external and internal evaluations were manually reviewed by a team consisting of a research intern specializing in NLP and healthcare, a biostatistician, and a group of pediatric surgeons. All pediatric surgeons involved in the evaluation have over five years of clinical experience, and they routinely treat Congenital Diaphragmatic Hernia (CDH) patients, which provided valuable insights into the clinical relevance and accuracy of the assistant's responses.

The research intern and biostatistician were responsible for verifying the technical aspects of the assistant's responses, such as consistency in document retrieval and adherence to the prompt template, ensuring the system followed the intended workflow. Their expertise in natural language processing and statistical analysis helped ensure objectivity in evaluating the assistant's performance, even though they did not directly assess clinical accuracy.

To evaluate the responses from both the external and internal evaluations, the team manually checked both the retrieved documents and the generated answers, applying the following 3-level criteria:

- **Correct answer.** When the response is supported by the retrieved documents.
- **Correct no-answer.** When the assistant replies with something like "I'm afraid I don't know the answer," and the retrieved documents are, indeed, insufficient to form an accurate answer.
- **Incorrect answer.** When the answer is not supported by the retrieved documents or contradicts the information in them.

4   Results

4.1   RQ1: Evaluation of the Assistant's Medical Query Capabilities

Table 2 summarizes the assistant's baseline performance across five question categories from the preliminary internal evaluation. This assessment tested the assistant's basic ability to handle various queries, filter irrelevant ones, and focus on CDH. While useful for evaluating core functionality, again these results should be viewed cautiously due to the synthetic questions.

The assistant correctly handled all 100 difficult CDH, medically inappropriate, general pediatric, and non-medical questions. For the standard CDH questions, the assistant correctly answered 19 out of 100. Each correct answer included relevant supporting sources, which were verified for their relevance and directly addressed the questions. There were no incorrect answers, as the assistant correctly declined to answer the remaining 81 questions. The frequent declination to respond highlighted the need for expanding the CDH knowledge base. Although the evaluation offered useful insights into the assistant's ability to filter inappropriate and irrelevant queries, the results should be interpreted with caution due to the synthetic nature of the questions. This baseline is especially important because our assistant is designed to provide answers only if the information can be found in the documents included in the prompt (see Listing 1.1), rather than relying on the LLM's foundational knowledge, which we consider unreliable.

4.2 RQ2: External Evaluation Results

We analyzed logs from the external evaluation with 258 questions across 68 conversations. The healthcare professionals primarily asked standard CDH-related questions, and the types of questions differed from the synthetic ones used in the internal evaluation. This limited our ability to assess the assistant's performance on more complex or non-medical questions. Of the 258 questions, the assistant answered 67 (26%) correctly and declined to answer 189. It gave incorrect answers to two questions regarding the use of inhaled nitric oxide (iNO) for treating pulmonary hypertension in CDH patients, citing insufficiently supportive sources.

In contrast, during the internal evaluation, which used synthetic questions, the assistant correctly managed all difficult CDH, inappropriate, general pediatric, and non-medical questions by declining to answer where appropriate. For standard CDH-related questions, the assistant answered 19 out of 100 correctly, with relevant supporting sources. There were no incorrect responses, but it declined to answer the remaining 81 questions, highlighting the need to expand the CDH knowledge base. Additionally, the physicians in the external evaluation did not ask the same variety of questions as those in the internal evaluation, further complicating the comparison between the two settings.

Table 2. Baseline Assistant Performance in Preliminary Query Evaluation

Question Category	Correct Answers	Correct No-answers	Incorrect Answers
Standard CDH Questions	19%	81%	0%
Complex CDH Questions	0%	100%	0%
Unethical Questions about CDH	0%	100%	0%
General Pediatric Medical Questions	0%	100%	0%
Non-Medically Related Questions	0%	100%	0%

4.3   RQ3: Identification of Knowledge Gaps in the CDH Assistant

To identify specific knowledge gaps in the assistant's responses, we conducted an analysis of both synthetically generated questions and those posed by medical professionals using LDA (Latent Dirichlet Allocation). The topic modeling process identified 13 distinct topics related to CDH, with a coherence score of 0.98, indicating a strong consistency and relevance among the topics. We subsequently assessed the assistant's performance within these topics, evaluating the proportion of correctly answered questions. Table 3 provides a detailed breakdown of the assistant's performance across these 13 topics, using N/M to denote the number of questions answered correctly (N) out of the total questions posed (M) in each topic.

For the synthetic questions, the assistant exhibited strong performance only in the Surgical Outcomes and Hernia-Related Procedures category, successfully answering all 13 questions. However, significant knowledge gaps were evident in several areas, not limited to Diagnosis and Severity $(0/26)$, Cardiac Support and Surgery Complications $(0/18)$, and Echocardiography and Respiratory Complications $(0/6)$. Overall, the assistant answered 19 out of 100 synthetic questions correctly, yielding a performance rate of 19%.

In contrast, the assistant's performance on questions posed by medical professionals was more evenly distributed, although clear gaps remained in areas such as Fetal Interventions and Outcomes $(0/6)$, Pediatric Management and Challenges $(0/1)$, and Aortic Issues and Management $(0/3)$. Overall, it answered 67 out of 258 questions from medical professionals, resulting in a performance rate of 26%. Cumulatively, the assistant achieved an overall performance rate of 24%, correctly answering 86 out of 358 questions. Based on the findings, it is recommended that future versions of the assistant focus on targeted training in areas with identified knowledge gaps, particularly where no correct answers were given. An automated LDA-driven approach to identifying and updating the knowledge base with those gaps will improve the assistant's ability to handle complex medical inquiries and provide healthcare professionals with up-to-date information.

4.4   RQ4: Performance Reevaluation After Knowledge Base Update

Based on the poor results in Table 3, we expanded the assistant's knowledge base with the help of a research librarian from St. Joseph's Hospital in Orange County. She conducted a PubMed search using queries such as "Congenital Diaphragmatic Hernia $< topic >$," where $< topic >$ was replaced with specific topics from Table 3 (e.g., "Aortic Issues and Management" or "Pediatric Management and Challenges"). This search resulted in 770 additional papers. After updating the knowledge base, we reran the queries and re-evaluated the assistant's performance using the same criteria outlined in Sect. 3.4.

The results, shown in Table 5, demonstrate significant improvement. The assistant, which previously had 81 unanswered synthetic questions, was now

Table 3. Knowledge across different CDH Related Topics

Topic	Synthetic Questions	User Questions
Hernia Types and Imaging Advantages	0/1	2/14
Fetal Interventions and Outcomes	0/3	0/6
Echocardiography and Respiratory Complications	0/6	4/12
Diagnosis and Severity	0/26	30/98
Cardiac Support and Surgery Complications	0/18	4/29
Patient Care and Surgery	2/6	10/27
Pediatric Management and Challenges	0/2	0/1
Surgical Outcomes and Hernia-Related Procedures	13/13	5/25
Nutritional and Community Support	0/2	2/9
Fetal Diagnosis and Imaging	0/2	1/ 5
Pulmonary Hypertension and Repair Complications	4/14	8/24
Prenatal Indicators and Diagnosis	0/5	1/5
Aortic Issues and Management	0/2	0/3
Total	**19/100**	**67/258**

able to correctly answer 91 of them, leaving only 9 unanswered, resulting in a 91% success rate. Notably, there were still no incorrect answers.

In the user questions, the assistant's performance improved significantly, with its score increasing from 26% to 86.82% correct answers—a percentage that is on par with the synthetic questions. It had 12.40% no-answers. Somewhat surprisingly, there were two incorrect answers. One of the questions the assistant got wrong again was: "Explain the rationale behind the use of inhaled nitric oxide (iNO) at CHOC for managing pulmonary hypertension in patients with Congenital Diaphragmatic Hernia (CDH), focusing on its physiological effects as they relate to echocardiography findings and respiratory complications," from the Echocardiography and Respiratory Complications category. Another new question the assistant previously declined to answer but then answered incorrectly was: "What factors determine the problematic use of iNO in babies with severe CDH and left ventricular diastolic dysfunction at CHOC?" from the Pulmonary Hypertension and Repair Complications category.

For each of these questions, the assistant provided an answer with a source. Even though the answers are understandable, there is nowhere in these documents that includes evidence of why inhaled nitric oxide (iNO) is used at CHOC or the criteria at CHOC for using Prostaglandin E (PGE) in CDH patients with pulmonary hypertension (PH). Despite lacking sufficient knowledge on these topics, the assistant attempted to answer these questions confidently. In Table 4, we present the performance update with the revised knowledge base and showcase the performance in each of the CDH expected categories.

5   Discussion

Our evaluation demonstrates the assistant's potential to provide evidence-based answers for Congenital Diaphragmatic Hernia (CDH) using the latest research.

Table 4. Knowledge across different topics after knowledge base expansion

Topic	Synthetic Questions	User Questions
Hernia Types and Imaging Advantages	1/1	13/14
Fetal Interventions and Outcomes	3/3	6/6
Echocardiography and Respiratory Complications	6/6	10/12
Diagnosis and Severity	24/26	85/98
Cardiac Support and Surgery Complications	15/18	26/29
Patient Care and Surgery	6/6	25/27
Pediatric Management and Challenges	1/2	1/1
Surgical Outcomes and Hernia-Related Procedures	13/13	22/25
Nutritional and Community Support	1/2	8/9
Fetal Diagnosis and Imaging	2/2	2/ 5
Pulmonary Hypertension and Repair Complications	14/14	19/24
Prenatal Indicators and Diagnosis	5/5	4/5
Aortic Issues and Management	0/2	3/3
Total	**91/100**	**224/258**

Table 5. Assistant's Performance with Expanded Knowledge Base

	Correct Answers	Correct No-answers	Incorrect Answers
Synthetic Questions	91%	9%	0%
User Questions	86.82%	12.40%	0.78%

The assistant effectively addressed a wide range of queries, including complex CDH-related questions, medically inappropriate inquiries, general pediatric topics, and non-medical issues. It consistently adhered to the prompt instructions, only providing answers when its knowledge base contained the necessary information. Notably, it correctly declined to answer 81 out of 100 synthetic CDH questions, responding with, "I'm afraid I don't know the answer," when lacking sufficient information.

However, the user-submitted questions focused narrowly on specific CDH scenarios, such as "When do you refer a fetus with CDH to a fetal center?" and "How does prenatal diagnosis impact CDH management and outcomes?" While these questions allowed us to evaluate the assistant's ability to provide specialized medical advice, they did not test its performance on inappropriate or non-relevant queries. This limitation highlights the need for a more diverse set of evaluation questions to better assess the assistant's capabilities in real-world scenarios.

A notable concern from the external evaluation was the assistant's incorrect responses to two CDH-specific questions about inhaled nitric oxide (iNO) and Prostaglandin E at CHOC, despite lacking information on CHOC's practices. This underscores the need for improved uncertainty handling, where the assistant should express uncertainty or recommend consulting a healthcare professional when lacking sufficient knowledge. Enhancing these mechanisms will prevent incorrect answers and improve the assistant's reliability, particularly in high-stakes medical environments.

One of the most significant findings is the impact of regularly updating the knowledge base. By adding 770 new papers, we observed a substantial improvement in the assistant's performance. The internal evaluation score increased from $19/100$ to $91/100$, and the external evaluation score rose from $67/258$ to $224/258$. These results emphasize the importance of continuous knowledge base updates to maintain the accuracy and relevance of the assistant's responses.

The assistant shows great potential in delivering evidence-based care recommendations for CDH using the latest research findings. This capability could lead to wider adoption by healthcare practitioners, potentially improving patient outcomes and reducing variability in mortality rates. However, further evaluation is necessary to confirm its effectiveness and reliability in real-world settings. Future evaluations should include a broader range of user-submitted questions, including inappropriate and non-relevant ones, to thoroughly assess the assistant's performance across diverse contexts and challenges.

6   Limitations

Our study has several limitations to acknowledge. First, we used Google Surveys to gather feedback on the assistant but received responses from only eight users because the survey was blocked on hospital computers. This small number of responses limited our ability to evaluate the assistant's performance from a qualitative perspective. Additionally, the external evaluation included only CDH-related questions, which means the findings may not apply to other medical topics, limiting the generalizability of our results.

In the internal evaluation, 80% of CDH questions were generated using ChatGPT-4 due to limited physician-provided questions, which may have introduced bias. Since the synthetic questions were created by the same model that powers the assistant, it likely improved the assistant's accuracy, as the questions shared similar language and structure with its training. However, real-world clinician questions are more varied and complex, making them more challenging for the assistant. Even with CDH expert reviews, synthetic questions may not reflect real scenarios. Future evaluations will use more physician-generated questions to assess the assistant.

7   Conclusion

We developed a RAG-based medical assistant using GPT-4 for CDH questions. Initial evaluations showed the assistant answered only 19 of 100 synthetic questions correctly but effectively filtered out inappropriate queries. In an external evaluation, it responded correctly to 67 out of 258 questions from healthcare professionals. After expanding the knowledge base with 770 additional papers, its performance improved significantly, answering 91 of 100 internal and 224 of 258 external questions. This highlights the importance of regular updates for accuracy and relevance. We also created a 250-question CDH dataset for future AI research.

Further evaluation with diverse real-world questions is needed to confirm the assistant's reliability in clinical scenarios, as real-world queries are more complex. Testing its ability to handle ethically challenging medical inquiries will be essential. Regular updates and improvements in managing uncertainty will be crucial for the assistant's ongoing accuracy and safe clinical deployment.

Acknowledgments. We thank the research computational science team at Children's Hospital of Orange County for their feedback, assistance, and ideas in improving this medical assistant.

Disclosure of Interests. The authors have no competing interests with this manuscript.

References

1. Thirunavukarasu, A.J., Ting, D., Elangovan, K., Gutierrez, L., Tan, T.F., Ting, D.: Large language models in medicine. Nat. Med. **29**(8), 1930–1940 (2023)
2. Zakka, C., et al.: Almanac-retrieval-augmented language models for clinical medicine. NEJM AI **1**(2), AIoa2300068 (2024)
3. Soong, D., et al.: Improving accuracy of gpt-3/4 results on biomedical data using a retrieval-augmented language model. arXiv preprint arXiv:2305.17116 (2023)
4. Jin, M., et al.: Health-llm: Personalized retrieval-augmented disease prediction model. arXiv preprint arXiv:2402.00746 (2024)
5. Lozano, A., Fleming, S.L., Chiang, C.C., Shah, N.: Clinfo. ai: an open-source retrieval-augmented large language model system for answering medical questions using scientific literature. In: Pacific Symposium on BiocomputinG 2024, pp. 8–23. World Scientific (2023)
6. Wu, K., et al.: How well do llms cite relevant medical references? an evaluation framework and analyses. arXiv preprint arXiv:2402.02008 (2024)
7. Ferber, D., et al.: Gpt-4 for information retrieval and comparison of medical oncology guidelines. NEJM AI **1**(6), AIcs2300235 (2024)
8. Achiam, J., et al.: Gpt-4 technical report. arXiv preprint arXiv:2303.08774 (2023)
9. Tonmoy, S., Zaman, S., Jain, V., Rani, A., Rawte, V., Chadha, A., Das, A.: A comprehensive survey of hallucination mitigation techniques in large language models. arXiv preprint arXiv:2401.01313 (2024)
10. Lewis, P., et al.: Retrieval-augmented generation for knowledge-intensive nlp tasks. Adv. Neural Inform. Process. Syst. **33**, 9459–9474 (2020)
11. Guner, Y.S., Harting, M.T., Jancelewicz, T., Peter, T.Y., Di Nardo, M., Nguyen, D.V.: Variation across centers in standardized mortality ratios for congenital diaphragmatic hernia receiving extracorporeal life support. J. Pediatr. Surg. **57**(11), 606–613 (2022)
12. Douze, M., et al.: The faiss library (2024)
13. Shanahan, M., McDonell, K., Reynolds, L.: Role play with large language models. Nature **623**(7987), 493–498 (2023)
14. Blei, D.M., Ng, A.Y., Jordan, M.I.: Latent dirichlet allocation. J. Mach. Learn. Res. **3**, 993–1022 (2003)

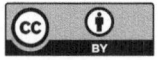

Identification of Molecular Leads for Treatment of Secondary TBI via Analysis of Gene Expression in Models of Traumatic Brain Injury in Combination with Two-Dimensional and Three-Dimensional Drug Library Analysis

Sarah Randall[1,2(✉)] ⓘ, Andreina Giron[1,3] ⓘ, Zoe Flyer[1] ⓘ, Alice Martino[1] ⓘ, and John Schomberg[1,3] ⓘ

[1] Children's Hospital of Orange County, Orange, CA 92868, USA
srandall02@icloud.com
[2] Biola University, La Mirada, CA 90639, USA
[3] University of California, Irvine, CA 92697, USA

Abstract. Traumatic brain injury (TBI) is a common and serious clinical problem with high variability in injury severity. Current clinical therapies generally only manage downstream effects of TBI. Thus, there is an increasing interest in finding treatments that can directly address underlying physiological responses such as edema, cell apoptosis, and tissue oxidation. We applied open-source, clinician-accessible informatics methods that identified differentially expressed genes (DEGs) in curated TBI rodent models, found associated hub genes and genetic pathways, and determined novel chemical leads for treatments that target key pathways associated with secondary inflammatory injury in TBI. Differential expression analysis was performed by identifying DEGs between models of TBI and controls. Pathway analysis was completed to determine the up and down regulated genes enriched in each gene pathway and to delineate DEGs in post TBI models over a 48-h recovery period. A molecular similarity search using over 22,000 known molecules was then run against the identified ligands. The pathways determined to be relevant to secondary TBI were inflammation, oxidative stress, cell apoptosis, and angiogenesis, a marker for blood-brain barrier permeability. The similarity search yielded 95 potential ligand matches found in PubChem's database. 20 ligands were determined to have potential in neuropathological treatment research or were associated with gene pathways relevant to TBI. The methodology reported in this study can be applied to other gene expression datasets to enable clinicians to identify viable treatment leads in rare or neglected diseases.

Keywords: cheminformatics · bioinformatics · traumatic brain injury · differential expression

---

The original version of the chapter has been revised. The order of authors has been corrected. A correction to this chapter can be found at https://doi.org/10.1007/978-3-031-88346-0_6

L. Ehwerhemuepha et al. (Eds.): IPLDSC 2024, CCIS 2386, pp. 47–71, 2025.
https://doi.org/10.1007/978-3-031-88346-0_4

1 Introduction

Traumatic brain injury (TBI) is a common and serious clinical problem globally with injury types ranging from a simple blow to the head to a penetrating injury to the brain. As the leading cause of death and disability among young people in developed countries, it is estimated that approximately 57 million people worldwide have been hospitalized following TBI [1]. In the United States, TBI accounts for 2.5 million visits to the Emergency Department and contributes to 50,000 deaths annually [2]. Young infants, adolescents between ages 15 and 19, and adults aged 65 and older are among the most at risk of sustaining a traumatic brain injury [3]. TBI has also drawn more attention for its adverse neuropsychological outcomes for military personnel [4] and athletes who play contact sports due to their increased propensity for reinjury, cognitive slowing, early onset Alzheimer's, and chronic traumatic encephalopathy [5].

Damage to the brain after a TBI is sustained can be separated into primary injury and secondary injury. Primary injury is instantaneous damage to the brain, causing bleeding, nerve damage, blood clots, leading to seizures stroke, coma, and infections in the brain. Secondary injury refers to the subsequent damage that occurs over hours to days due to altered cerebral blood flow and inflammatory processes such as vasospasm and increased intracranial pressure, causing long-term physical, cognitive, and behavioral impairments such as insomnia, cognitive decline, and posttraumatic depression [6]. On the cellular and molecular level, brain swelling caused by primary TBI occurs due to the failure of membrane transporters and leakage of the blood–brain barrier (BBB), resulting in a combination of cytotoxic, ionic, and vasogenic edema. After the initial injury, a cascade of gene functions set off an inflammatory response which ignites the secondary phase of the disease course causing edema, cell apoptosis, and tissue oxidation, known as secondary brain injury. Without immediate treatment, morbidity and mortality rates due to secondary TBI increase dramatically [7]. Current clinical therapies such as decompressive craniectomy and osmotherapy manage downstream effects of primary TBI but do not halt the underlying molecular cascade leading to brain swelling and further damage leading to secondary TBI [8]. Additionally, there is no drug for mediating secondary brain injury that has been approved by the Food and Drug administration (FDA) [9]. However, with advances in the understanding of the molecular underpinnings of TBI, newer targeted therapeutics may help with further improvement in survival and reduction in disability in patients with brain swelling.

Research has been done using adult rat models to facilitate the investigation of new noninvasive methods to mitigate the downstream effects of TBI [10]. Different modes of TBI induction such as unilateral controlled cortical impact (CCI) or lateral moderate fluid percussion are used to induce TBI in animal models and gene expression levels in brain tissue are then measured from those experiments. RNA sequencing is then conducted to determine which genes, pathways and networks are significantly altered by the initial impact, and the following physiological response. Previous studies on TBI have involved attempts to elucidate the temporal sequence of events after the initial injury by analyzing multiple mechanisms related to the occurrence of apoptosis and its relationship to inflammation in adult rat models [11]. Further evidence shows that prostaglandin (PG) synthases and cyclooxygenase (COX) 1 and 2 may contribute to secondary neurodegeneration, which is closely associated with neuroinflammation

[12]. Other studies have taken further steps to identify more potential target genes using genome-wide RNA-sequencing and have identified compounds that showed a strong connectivity with TBI signals in neuronal cell lines that reverse pathologic gene expression or reinforce the expression of recovery-related genes [13]. Bioinformatic analysis on microarray data in TBI experiments has also helped identify key molecular pathways and networks associated with post-TBI neural injury [14].

Collections of these and other annotated and curated experiments on TBI in the Gene Expression Omnibus database (GEO) provide sufficient data that allow for a comprehensive analysis, which can inform the identification of novel molecular leads. These experiments have not yet been aggregated and analyzed in conjunction with each other, adjusting for differences between datasets. Using results of the gene expression output, conclusions about which genes should be targeted can be drawn using information about the enrichment of differentially expressed genes within pathways regulating physical and metabolic processes pertinent to recovery from neurologic injury. Here, we perform analysis on aggregated data reported in recent TBI studies examining gene expression in rodent models, by finding known ligands that bind to genes significantly enriched within the pathways associated with secondary neurologic injury. In this study we describe open source, clinician accessible informatics methods used to identify differentially expressed genes in curated TBI mouse models, identify critical genes and genetic pathways based upon gene expression output results, and determine novel chemical leads for treatments that target key pathways associated with secondary inflammatory injury in TBI. Our goal is to utilize fully open-source genomic and cheminformatic tools to identify hub genes that are most directly associated with neurological damage post-injury and find small molecules with known repressive interactions to control abnormal gene expression levels in reaction to TBI. The methodology reported in this study can be further applied to other gene expression datasets to enable clinicians to identify viable treatment leads in rare or neglected diseases.

2 Methods

2.1 Data Sources

All TBI experiment data were collected from the Gene Expression Omnibus (GEO). GEO is an international public repository that archives and freely distributes microarray, next-generation sequencing, and other forms of high-throughput functional genomics data submitted by the research community. Five distinct gene expression datasets were collected from the GEO database to compare differences pertaining to the method of TBI induction (GSE23653, GSE24047, GSE45997, GSE67836, and GSE111452-GPL22740). These datasets were chosen from GEO using filters of neurological trauma, brain injury, head injury, in rodent (*rattus norwegicus*) models of TBI with 6 or more models within an experiment to ensure sufficient statistical power for identifying differentially expressed genes (DEGs). This threshold was set to allow for robust comparison across conditions and to minimize the risk of false positives, enhancing the reliability of the results. Additionally, by including multiple studies, we aimed to capture a broader sample of genes, thereby enabling a more comprehensive and reliable pooling of results, which enhances the exportability of these results. All initial RNA sequencing analysis to determine gene up/downregulation was performed by the respective authors and researchers of each experiment.

2.2   Differentially Expressed Gene (DEG) Analysis

Analyzed differentially expressed genes (DEGs) from expression datasets come from both *in vitro* and *in vivo* models. GSE2365 is an *in vitro* DNA microarray study that includes expression data on mature cortical neuronal clusters maintained 24 h following complete axonal severance [15]. GSE24047 datasets utilized brain samples from the cerebral cortex of rats subjected to TBI model of lateral moderate fluid percussion injury (FPI) in an effort to examine the levels of gene expression in the early phase of traumatic brain injury. Since most critical DEGs impacted by TBI were seen emerging around 12 to 24 h post injury, we examined the expression data set at the 12-h time point when compared to other datasets GSE45997 used microarray analysis to determine which genes, pathways and networks were significantly altered in the ipsilateral and contralateral hemi-brain tissue in adult rats after receiving a unilateral CCI [11]. Gene expression data for ipsilateral and contralateral hemi-brain tissue were compared against each other and the other three TBI experimental datasets. Lateral fluid percussion injury and head acceleration rotational injury rat models of trauma induction were used in GSE67836 to evaluate gene expression profiles in the frontal cortex at 1 month when secondary damage could be detected [16]. GSE111452-GPL2270 is an extended study on acute TBI characterizing the temporal genomic profile of injured cortex brain tissue up to 12 months post-TBI under the fluid percussion TBI model. Only gene expression data at hour 24 was included for this analysis [17].

2.3   Gene Annotation Tools and Sources

Differential expression was performed on the genes listed in each dataset using the GEO2R functionality within GEO. GEO2R is an interactive web tool that allows users to compare two or more groups of samples in a GEO Series to identify differentially expressed genes (DEGs) across experimental conditions [18]. R packages EdgeR and Limma within R 4.3.1 were used for analysis of datasets. Selection criteria for DEGs from GEO2R included genes whose Log2 fold expression change was greater than 2.00 or less than -2.00, the standard cutoff for change in expression, with p-value < 0.05 [19]. The number of significantly upregulated or downregulated DEGs shared between each of the five expression datasets was counted in order to infer the degree of relatedness between genes affected by different modes of TBI. A similar numeric comparison was done for GSE24047 within the 3-, 6-, 12-, and 48-h datasets and gene names and associated pathways were documented.

The Reactome Pathway Analysis tool was used for pathway analysis on the DEGs. Reactome is an open-source, open access, manually curated and peer-reviewed pathway database that allows users to submit genes to determine which pathways are enriched with certain genes [20]. Criteria for selection included pathways with p-value and false discovery rate (FDR) < 0.05. Gene annotation was reviewed within the STRING database to search for the most influential genes responsible for inciting secondary TBI injury.

STRING is a database that contains gene annotations and allows for visualization of known and predicted protein-protein interactions [21]. Criteria for gene review were based on experimental evidence, topology and gene pathway hierarchy, and the relevancy of annotation within affect pathways, allowing us to find influential genes based upon the number of connections a gene has within a genetic pathway that have been validated through experimental results.

2.4 Cheminformatic Analysis

Ligands for DEGs were evaluated and selected using the Research Collaboratory for Structural Bioinformatics Protein Data Bank (RCSB PDB). RCSB PDB is the US data center for the global Protein Data Bank archive of 3D structure data for large biological molecules (proteins, DNA, and RNA) in fundamental biology, health, energy, and biotechnology [22]. PubChem's structure similarity search tool was used to generate a list of similarly structured ligands for each gene identified to compare to PubChem's official database of documented drugs and chemicals. PubChem is an open-source chemistry database at the National Institutes of Health (NIH) that contains information on chemical and physical properties of small molecules such as biological activities, safety, and toxicity data [23]. Similarity was determined using the 2D simplified molecular-input line-entry system (SMILES) and 3D structure of each ligand. A Tanimoto similarity score of 85% was used as a threshold to exclude molecular matches with low similarity [24]. The Lipinski rule of five was used as the filter criteria in the structure similarity search tool for ligands to be included in the comparison. After completing the comparison, a phylogenetic approach to chemical analysis was done to organize the molecular matches into leading phylogram clusters based on functionality and structure. Annotation within clusters and found chemicals was performed to organize and classify the chemicals into functional families.

A final literature search into each of the matched chemicals was done to evaluate whether these treatments were used in TBI, or other treatment related to neurodegenerative diseases and validate the use of these molecules and treatment methods. Guidelines for measuring strength of literature evidence favored molecules that met toxicity criteria, had evidence of medicinal properties, and had been used in either clinical trials, in vivo rat models, or in vitro cell lines. Literature defining experimental use of drug molecules must also have shown capability of positively affecting pathways relevant to TBI or be used with the intent to treat related neurological damage.

3 Results

3.1 Commonly Expressed TBI Genes Among Separate Experimental Gene Expression Datasets

A numerical comparison of affected DEGs showed some degree of overlap between separate gene expression datasets (Fig. 1). The two datasets with the greatest number of overlapping DEGs occur between GSE45997_ipsilateral and GSE45997_contralateral. Between two separate experiments, most DEG overlap occurs between GSE24047 and GSE45997_ipsilateral with 32 shared DEGs. There are four cases where DEGs were shared across 3 datasets: 5 DEGs were found in common with GSE24047, GSE45997_ipsilateral, and GSE45997_contralateral, 4 DEGs between GSE23653, GSE45997_contralateral, and GSE45997_ipsilateral, 2 DEGs between GSE24047, GSE23653, and GSE45997_ipsilateral, and another 2 DEGs in common between GSE111452, GSE45997_contralateral, and GSE45997_ipsilateral. There were no instances found in which DEGs were shared across more than 3 experiments.

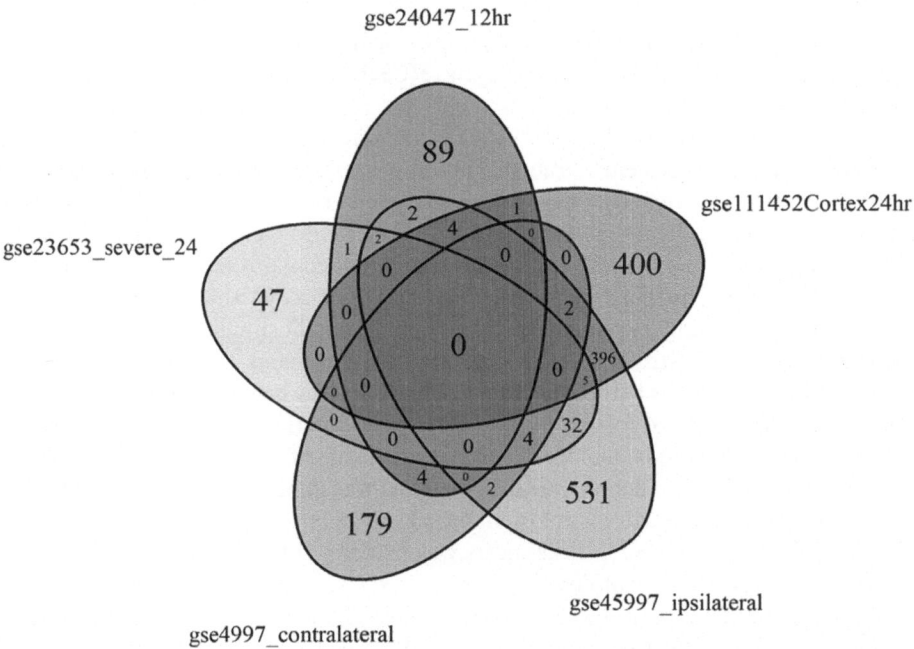

Fig. 1. Diagram showing the number of significantly affected genes shared among 5 separate TBI experimental datasets from GEO. Color key: Blue = GSE23653_severe_24hr (In vitro neurons). Purple = GSE45997 (Contralateral). Green = GSE45997 (Ipsilateral). Orange = GSE111452_24hr (Cerebral cortex). Yellow = GSE24047_12hr (Cerebral cortex).

Gene markers for apoptosis (*Hspb1*) and cell proliferation (*Gbp2*) were commonly shared between datasets GSE2365, GSE24047, and GSE45997_ipsilateral. Some DEGs directly related to acute inflammatory pathways (*Stat3, Lbp, Serpina3n, Tmbim1*) were also shared between at least 3 datasets where GSE24047 is included. Other DEGs shared between 3 datasets are involved in apoptosis and inflammatory responses (*Stat3, Lcn2, Tmbim1*) and oxidative stress (*Cp*). Apart from shared DEGs, many regulatory genes affected by TBI were identified within inflammatory and apoptotic pathways. These DEGs are highlighted particularly in the GSE24047 and GSE45997_ipsilateral datasets (Table 1). DEGs involved in inflammatory response include modulators of interleukin and cytokine signaling and pyroptosis. Genes such as *Stat3, Casp4, and Grb2* were also seen as shared between other expression datasets.

Table 1. List of regulatory hub DEGs found within TBI gene expression datasets and grouped by pathway. Gene function and pathways verified using Reactome and STRING documentation (FDR < 0.05, p-value < 0.05).

Experiment Name	Pathway	Hub Genes
GSE24047_12 h	Interleukin-10 signaling	*Ilb1, Il1r2, Stat3*
GSE24047_12 h	Signaling by Interleukins	*Cebpd, Il1r2, Stat3, Ilb1*
GSE24047_12 h	Cytokine Signaling in Immune system	*Fos, Cebpd, Irf1, Il1r2, Stat3,*
GSE24047_12 h	Interleukin-4 and Interleukin-13 signaling	*Fos, Cebpd, Stat3*
GSE24047_12 h	Immune System	*Casp4, Irf1, Il1b*
GSE24047_12 h	Chemokine receptors bind chemokines	*Irf1*
GSE24047_12 h	Interferon Signaling	*Irf1*
GSE24047_12 h	Pyroptosis	*Casp4, Irf1, Il1b*
GSE24047_12 h	CLEC7A/inflammasome pathway	*Il1b*
GSE45997_ipsilateral	Interleukin-4 and Interleukin-13 signaling	*Socs3, Il6, Cebpd, Stat3*
GSE45997_ipsilateral	Interleukin-10 signaling	*Il6, Cebpd, Stat3, Il1b, Ccl2*
GSE45997_ipsilateral	Signaling by Interleukins	*Grb2, Pik3r3, Stat3, Il6, Casp3, App, Socs3, Timp1*

3.2 Gene Pathways Within Lateral-Fluid Percussion Time Point Experiment GSE24047

Comparison of the number of upregulated and downregulated DEGs (log(FC) ± 2.00) common between each timepoint shows there are multiple concurrent DEGs that show up throughout the 48-h observation period (Fig. 2). About 14 concurrent DEGs are active at 3, 6 and 12 h post-injury, and the majority of DEGs are observed 6 h after initial injury. More unique genes are seen in later TBI stages, especially at the 48-h time point as reflected by fewer active DEGs in common with earlier stages. There were also no active DEGs that were seen in all 4 timepoints.

Analysis of specific DEGs within each GSE24047 data allowed for mapping specific genes to their respective pathways at the time expression was measured (Table 2). At each time point, a different gene pathway is highlighted by the genes that are the most upregulated within that pathway. Inflammatory genes related to chemokine signaling immune response and interleukin inflammatory markers (*Il1b, Il1a, Tnfaip3, Il1r2*) were the most upregulated in the 3rd hour post-injury. The 6th hour shows a continued increased upregulation of inflammatory markers seen at hour 3 and present new upregulated genes related to oxidative stress (*Hmox1*), apoptosis (*Myc, Birc3*), and BBB disruption (*Lcn2*). Hour 12 showed an upregulation of new inflammatory genes (*Cebpd,*

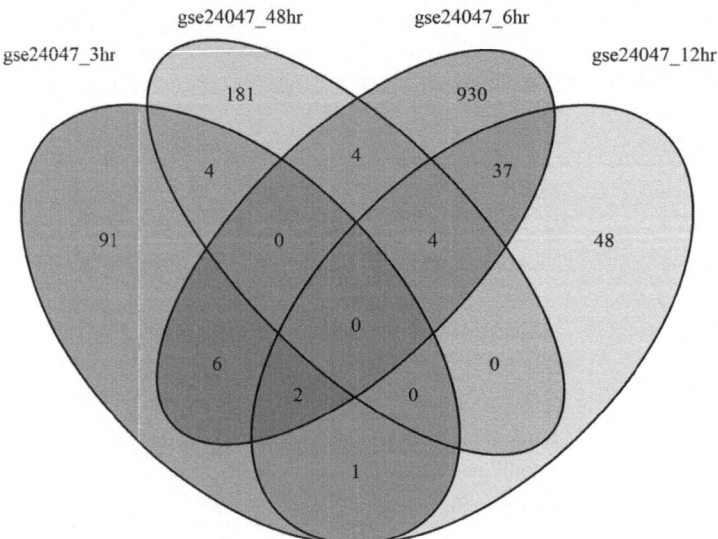

Fig. 2. Diagram showing the number of significantly affected DEGs within each timepoint (3-h, 6-h, 12-h, and 48-h) following Shojo's lateral fluid percussion injury in the rat brain. Data taken from GEO experiment GSE24047.

Irgm2), while some inflammatory genes begin to stabilize (*Il1b*) or become downregulated (*Lbp*). Both the oxidative stress and angiogenesis pathways from Hour 6 continue to be upregulated into the 12th hour along with genes related to cell apoptosis. By the 48th hour, inflammatory response to TBI has become faint. Most expression data of previously seen inflammatory markers and signs of damage were not recorded except for *Lcn2* and *Lgals3*. Signs of tissue amelioration included the downregulation of genes related to cell apoptosis (*Lcn2*) and the upregulation of antioxidant gene pathway expression (*Arl11*). Based on this analysis, we were able to construct a timeline summarizing which gene pathways are highlighted at each timepoint over the 48-h recovery period (Fig. 3).

3.3 Ligand Matches for Gene Pathways

The ligand search in the RCSB PDB yielded 19 unique ligands, all of which have experimentally determined interactions with TBI relevant genes found in the time point and cross-experimental analyses (Table 3, Appendix 1). A subsequent molecule structure similarity search across over 22,000 known molecules run against the identified ligands yielded 95 small molecule matches found in PubChem's database (Appendix 2). Phylogenetic chemical analysis shows that the 95 small molecule matches can be grouped into 8 distinct chemical groups, some of which contain anti-inflammatory properties (Fig. 4). Out of the original 95 small molecule matches, 20 molecules were determined to be relevant in neuropathological treatment research or addressed gene pathways relevant to TBI after further literature review (Table 4).

Table 2. TBI Relevant Genes in GSE24047 experiment with log fold change expression of relevant TBI genes in experiment GSE24047. Gene function and pathways verified using STRING documentation.

Inflammation		Oxidative stress		Apoptosis		Angiogenesis	
Genes	logFC	Genes	logFC	Genes	logFC	Genes	logFC
3-hr		3-hr		3-hr		3-hr	
Il1a	5.73	Nfkbiz	3.12	Bcl2a1	3.02	Adamts1	2.08
Il1b	5.06	Gbp2	2.39	Fosb	2.29	6-hr	
Il6	3.08	Bcl2a1	3.02	Tfpi2	2.59	Sele	4.35
Tnfaip3	2.79	Adamts1	2.08	Egr2	2.13	Adamts1	3.31
Irf1	2.31	6-hr		6-hr		12-hr	
Tnf	2.06	Hmox1	2.32	Tlr2	2.1	Sele	3.25
6-hr		Myc	2.27	Ifit3	2.24	Serpine1	3.4
Slpi	2.41	Birc3	2.19	S100a9	5.96	Adamts1	3.55
Tnfaip3	3.25	Lcn2	4.24	Gadd45g	2.99		
Irf1	2.83	Nfkbiz	2.17	Fos	2.04		
Cebpd	3.25	Gbp2	4.52	Tfpi2	3.56		
12-hr		Clec7a	2.1	Bcl2a1	3.39		
Slpi	4.51	Hspb1	3.03	12-hr			
Stat3	2.06	12-hr		S100a9	5.12		
Casp4	2.15	Lcn2	5.16	S100a8	4.1		
Il1b	2.67	Nfkbiz	2.03	Bcl2a1	2.81		
Irf1	2.81	Hspb1	4.44	Ifit3	2.26		
Il1r2	3.94	Gbp2	4.49	Fos	2.52		
Lbp	-2.21	48-hr		Tfpi2	3.56		
Cebpd	3.43	Lcn2	-3.83	Bcl2a1	3.39		
Irgm2	3.54			48-hr			
				Lgals3	-2.6		
				Arll1	2.33		

3.4 Literature Review of Known Molecules for Neuropathic Treatment

Recent investigations have been conducted to validate the potential use of identified molecules for treating neurodegenerative disorders and effects of neurological trauma. In vitro studies using bergapten, idebenone, and pinocembrin on cells have both been cited for their potential to attenuate inflammatory response specifically through the NLRP3 inflammasome pathway, which is closely tied with innate immune system response and associated with neurological damage [23–25]. Idebenone has also been used in in vivo neurological studies and has shown to lessen cerebral inflammatory injury in rat models caused by ischemic stroke [26]. Gallic acid can positively influence the cellular apoptotic

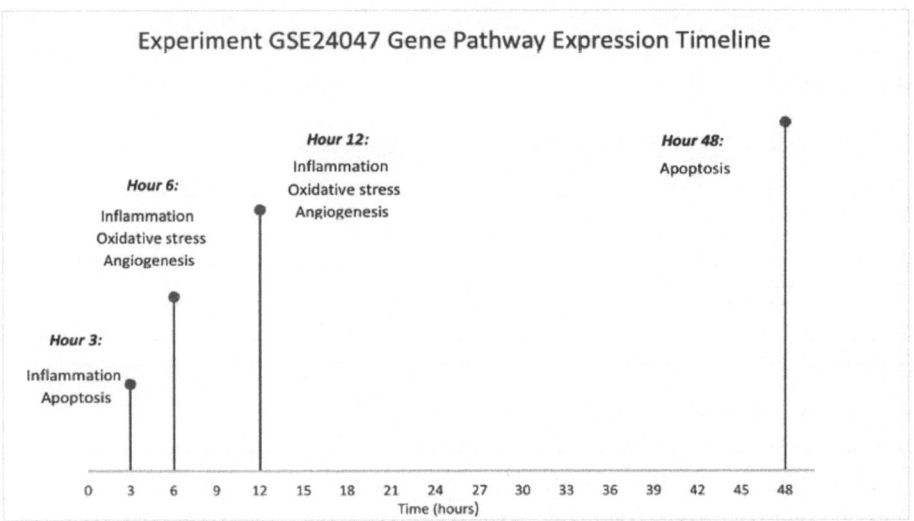

Fig. 3. Timeline depicting the pathways that are up and downregulated over the 48-h time period for experiment GSE24047.

pathway by inhibiting the anti-apoptotic protein BCL-2 while reducing expression of its eponymous gene, encouraging apoptosis, and elevating levels of antioxidant enzymes in cancer research models [27].

Psoralen (CID 619) is a natural compound from which the compound 8-methoxypsoralen (8-MOP) and medication oxsoralen is derived from. Psoralen and its derivatives are approved and used globally to treat skin conditions including eczema, vitiligo, psoriasis, and palmoplantar pustulosis. Psoralen has also demonstrated medical efficacy in controlling pathologies in the immune, nervous, motor system, and cardio-vascular systems in modern medicine [28, 29]. Recent research has shown promise for using 8-MOP to treat the effects of TBI due to its anti-inflammatory, antioxidant and tissue-repairing abilities. 8-MOP administration to neural cells treated with lipopolysac-charide (LPS) induced inflammation and LPS-induced neuronal damage in microglia, as well as reducing neurological distress gene signals in *Cox2*, *Tlr4* by modulating the PPARγ/NF-κB pathway. Furthermore 8-MOP treatment for in vivo rat TBI models relieved neurological deficits, improved cognitive, learning and motor functions, and mitigated brain edema and neuroinflammation induced by TBI [30].

Paeonol, an extract of the plant *Paeonia albiflora*, manifests anti-inflammatory and antioxidative effects in multiple diseases. In one study for neuropathic pain treatment, namely chronic constriction injury (CCI), paeonol was found to significantly block neuroinflammation and astrocytic activation via blocking HDAC/miR-15a signaling. Expression of inflammatory genes such as *Tnf-α*, *Il-1β*, and *Il-6* were stabilized after administering paeonol in in vivo CCI rats [31]. Table 6 includes the R (CID 667495) and S (CID 932) enantiomers for naringenin, a bioflavonoid that can act against oxidative stress-induced neurobehavioral disorders and cognitive dysfunction in rodents based on a meta-analysis of twenty different studies. It was further shown that naringin can

Table 3. Ligands for identified TBI relevant genes matched by associated protein. All ligand abbreviations originate from RCSB PDB. See Appendix 1 for the official names of each ligand.

Experiment Name	Gene/Protein	Log2(FC)	P-value	RCSB Ligand Identifiers	Official Ligand Name(s)
GSE24047_12 h	STAT3	2.06	<0.001	KQV	Quinoline
GSE24047_12 h	FOS	2.31	<0.001	MV0	Methyl vanillate
GSE111452Cortex24 h	COX8A	23.23	0.003	CDL, HEA, PEE	Cardiolipin (CDL), Heme A (HEA), Phosphoethanolamine (PEE)
GSE111452Cortex24 h	COX6A1	28.04	0.002	CDL, HEA, PEE	Cardiolipin (CDL), Heme A (HEA), Phosphoethanolamine (PEE)
GSE111452Cortex24 h	COX6C	17.255	0.010	CDL, HEA, PEE, PLX, NDP, HEC, HEM, 8Q1, FMN	Cardiolipin (CDL), Heme A (HEA), Phosphoethanolamine (PEE), Pyridoxal Phosphate (PLX), NADP (NDP), Heme C (HEC), Hemin (HEM), Flavin Mononucleotide (FMN)
GSE111452Cortex24 h	ATP5D	5.37	0.002	CDL, 3PH	Cardiolipin (CDL), Phosphoenolpyruvate (3PH)
GSE111452Cortex24 h	NDUFB3	3.31	0.049	8Q1, CDL, PEE, PLX, FMN, HEA, HEC, HEM, NDP	8-Hydroxyquinoline (8Q1), Cardiolipin (CDL), Phosphoethanolamine (PEE), Pyridoxal Phosphate (PLX), Flavin Mononucleotide (FMN), Heme A (HEA), Heme C (HEC), Hemin (HEM), NADP (NDP)
GSE24047_3 h	TNF	2.06	<0.001	307	Threonine (307)
GSE24047_3 h	ICAM	2.05	<0.001	NAG	N-Acetyl-D-Glucosamine (NAG)
GSE24047_3 h	IL6	3.08	<0.001	NAG	N-Acetyl-D-Glucosamine (NAG)
GSE24047_3 h	IL1B	5.06	<0.001	NAG	N-Acetyl-D-Glucosamine (NAG)
GSE24047_3 h	TNFAIP3	2.79	<0.001	INN	Inosine (INN)
GSE24047_3 h	BCL2A1	3.02	< 0.001	CAD, K3Q	Cadaverine (CAD), Quinoline (K3Q)
GSE24047_6 h	TLR2	2.10	<0.001	NAG	N-Acetyl-D-Glucosamine (NAG)
GSE24047_6 h	IL1R2	3.26	0.005	NAG	N-Acetyl-D-Glucosamine (NAG)
GSE24047_6 h	SERPINE1	3.4	0.008	EMJ, GDE	Emodin (EMJ), Guanosine (GDE)

Phylogenetic Tree of Traumatic Brain Injury Treatment Lead Molecules

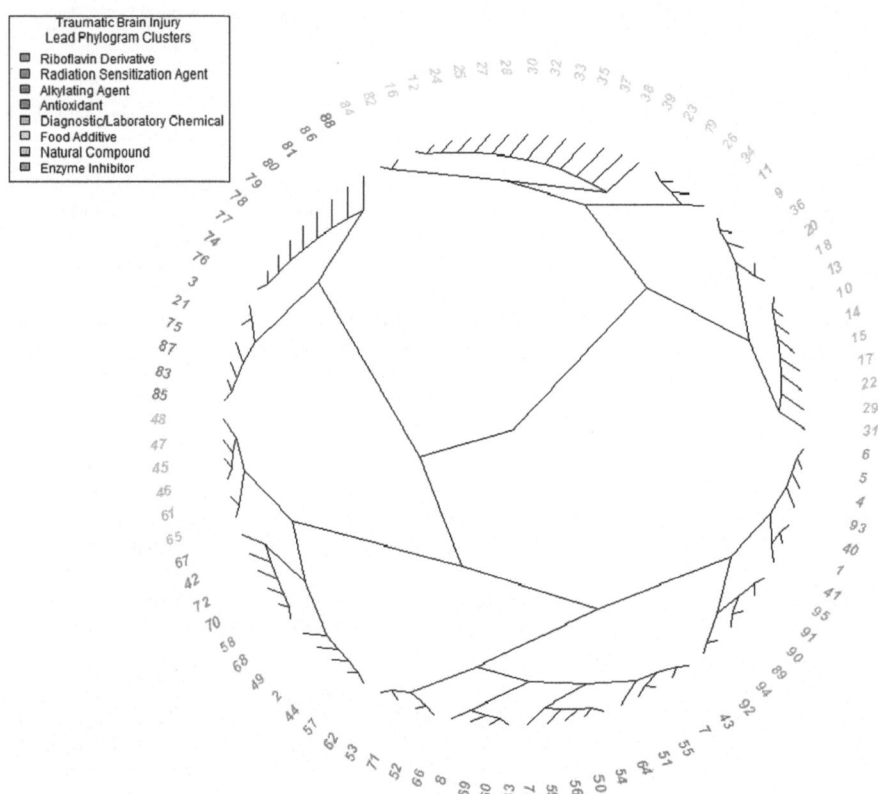

Fig. 4. Phylogenetic tree depicting relatedness among leading TBI molecule matches. See Appendix 2 for the 95 molecule matches referenced.

significantly restore the levels of common oxidative stress markers superoxide dismutase (SOD), catalase (CAT), glutathione-S-transferase (GST), reduced glutathione (GSH) ad lipid peroxidation (LPO) [32].

Table 4. List of the 20 small molecule matches with literature evidence of relevance in neuropathological treatment (Tanimoto Similarity Score > = 80%).

PubChem CID*	Chemical Name	Known Gene/Protein Interactions
3686	Idebenone	SERPINE1
493570	Riboflavin	COX6C, NDUFB3, NDUFB9, NDUFV1
4947	Propyl Gallate	SERPINE1
2355	Bergapten	Proto-oncogene C-FOS
10658	Angelicin	Proto-oncogene C-FOS
6199	Psoralen	Proto-oncogene C-FOS
60961	Adenosine	IL6, IL1B, ICAM, TLR2, IL1R2
370	Gallic acid	SERPINE1
5280961	Genistein	Proto-oncogene C-FOS
4114	Methoxsalen	Proto-oncogene C-FOS
114829	Liquiritigenin	Proto-oncogene C-FOS
68071	Pinocembrin	Proto-oncogene C-FOS
11092	Paeonol	Proto-oncogene C-FOS
10212	Pentosalen	Proto-oncogene C-FOS
5280443	Apigenin	Proto-oncogene C-FOS
667495	(2R)-5,7-dihydroxy-2-(4-hydroxyphenyl)-2,3-dihydro-4H-chromen-4-one	Proto-oncogene C-FOS
5318980	Icaritin	Proto-oncogene C-FOS
5281708	Daidzein	Proto-oncogene C-FOS
667495	(2R)-5,7-dihydroxy-2-(4-hydroxyphenyl)-2,3-dihydro-4H-chromen-4-one	Proto-oncogene C-FOS
932	5,7-Dihydroxy-2-(4-hydroxyphenyl)chroman-4-one	Proto-oncogene C-FOS

* PubChem CID is the compound identification number for each unique chemical structure in the PubChem database

Genistein, a flavonoid and nonsteroidal phytoestrogen found in soy, contains anti-inflammatory and neuroprotective effects with the ability to repair damage to the BBB [33]. The use of genistein has been evaluated as potential therapy in mice with TBI. It was found that two 15 mg/kg doses 24 h post-TBI showed a decrease in the development of brain edema and BBB permeability along with improved motor function in mice [34]. The natural polyphenol apigenin also contains BBB protective properties and targets multiple proteins and pathways similar to, or the same as those affected by TBI. Target proteins for apigenin show some parallel with upregulated proteins found in TBI rat models such as STAT3, COX2, CASP3, BCL2, and PTGS2. The use of apigenin has mostly been studied in ischemic stroke models, but studies have shown that apigenin has an inhibitory effect on multiple key proteins involving neurological inflammatory response and oxidative stress [35].

An intermediate product of riboflavin, flavin mononucleotide (FMN), has shown successful results in modulating LPS-induced neuroinflammation in microglial cells via anti-oxidative stress and anti-inflammation properties. Microglia have been cited as predominant contributors for neuroinflammation as resident immune cells, creating a significant risk factor for cognitive dysfunction. The mechanism by which FMN attenuates neuroinflammation is through modulation of the pro-inflammatory TNFR1/NF-κB signaling pathway in microglial cells. Zhang et al. established a biomimetic microglial nanoparticle strategy that is able to penetrate the BBB with enhanced microglial-targeted delivery efficiency; the result of which ameliorated cognitive impairment and dysfunctional synaptic plasticity in an LPS-induced inflammatory mouse model [36].

4 Discussion

In this study, we used fully open-source genomic and cheminformatic tools to identify hub genes that are most associated with secondary TBI and to find small molecules known to control abnormal gene expression levels. We began by looking at existing gene expression datasets to identify shared genes between different TBI experiments, then examined similarities and trends in one of the studies with expression data over a 48-h recovery period. The numerical comparison of upregulated and downregulated DEGs among separate gene expression datasets and within time point experiment GSE24047 showed similar degrees of overlap between gene expressions. Many regulatory DEGs involved in acute inflammatory response were highlighted in the GSE24047 experiment at the 3-, 6-, and 12-h marks. GSE45997_ipsilateral also corroborates several inflammatory DEGs found in GSE24047. GSE111452 datasets also included several of the identified dysregulated genes after TBI at 24-h in cortex tissue associated with acute phase response signaling and neuroinflammation. Along with genes from canonically associated acute inflammatory pathways, we searched to those that are strongly associated with the longer-term neurodegenerative effects such as oxidative stress, angiogenesis, and apoptosis to piece together a general depiction showing the approximate order in which these pathways become upregulated. As seen in Fig. 3, the inflammatory response pathway is predominant for the first 12–24 h after TBI. A few genes associated with oxidative stress and apoptosis begin to show increasing expression levels just within the first 3 h. Expression levels continue to worsen with new markers showing up until the 12th hour, where gene expression from all neurodegenerative pathways are at their highest. The majority of TBI markers appearing 12–24 h after injury appears to be consistent across each of these TBI data sets, highlighting a critical time window for clinical intervention. Most gene markers of brain damage have regressed 48 h after injury, yet neurological damage has already taken place. Many of these DEGs are known key hub genes in essential cell signaling pathways. Thus, these quantitative gene expression comparisons show that several regulatory genes listed in Table 1 and Table 2 are associated with acute inflammatory and immune response gene pathways [11, 15–37].

Many ligands from Table 3 show commonality in their effect on specific pathways, often matching with separate but intricately related proteins. For the ligand search, along with the key hub genes found in Table 1 and Table 2, we included genes that were not explicitly key regulatory genes yet showed astounding levels of upregulation. Such was the case for *Atp5d* and the *Cox* gene family which presented the highest log (FC) levels across multiple datasets. Despite not being key regulatory genes, their upregulation can still be noted for future pharmacological studies. Based on literature research and analysis of Supplemental Table 2 and Fig. 4, we found that the molecules with the strongest evidence and potential for use of treatment in neuropathology are riboflavin derivatives, antioxidants, and natural compounds. One listed molecule, adenine, is a notable exception. While not directly a treatment molecule, in that some experimental evidence shows that A_{2A} adenosine receptor antagonists applied to neurodegenerative conditions gives promising results, and the repurposing of ADP-activated $P2Y_{12}R$ antagonists toward neuroinflammation is being considered [38]. More research is needed to confirm these molecules for use in TBI models and patients.

This study has described the methodology for the use of public gene expression data found in GEO in conjunction with ligands identified through RCSPDB and PubChem to identify 198 novel treatment leads for secondary neurological injury in TBI patients. These leads were validated though a review of the literature for each lead that met filter criteria. Our methodology reported in this study can be further applied to other gene expression datasets to enable clinicians to identify viable treatment leads in rare or neglected diseases. Currently the pathway to drug development can take decades with new treatments taking over 10 years to develop on average [39]. Identifying publicly available software that can be utilized by physicians without bioinformatic training, or a research and development budget is a promising avenue in describing disease pathways and novel treatments for neglected diseases.

The limited number of treatment options for patients suffering from TBI is a testament to the lack of effective, safe, and affordable pharmaceuticals to control diseases that cause high mortality and morbidity [40]. The knowledge acquisition process leading to drug discovery can take years or decades of research before innovation can truly move forward. Thus, there is an increasing need for more expedient research methods to help accelerate research efforts in finding new treatments. Open-source research methodology utilizes public tools and datasets at no cost to identify treatment leads that meet toxicity and pharmacological activity criteria. Special knowledge is also not required, which is an invitation for physicians who can use their clinical expertise to spearhead the endeavor of knowledge acquisition for clinical and pharmaceutical research. Biomedical scientists and physicians who adapt open-source R&D methods can work together to make a significant difference in the drug development process for neglected diseases for which funds are limited. Therefore, an approach to cheminformatics such as the one outlined in our research is ideal for the identification of treatment leads when resources for in-vivo testing are limited.

Our accessible method of research also yielded results that provide evidence for common genes and pathways that are expressed across different types of injury mechanisms. Our pathway analyses depict the effects of TBI from two unique perspectives. The cross-experimental analysis highlighted genes in common among fluid percussion, weight drop, and rotational injury mechanisms, thus shedding light on which pathways to focus on. The time-point experiment analysis on GSE24047 supports the finding of similar pathogenic markers seen in other TBI studies further affirming our determination that the pathways leading to secondary TBI include inflammation, oxidative stress, cell apoptosis, and angiogenesis [41].

In summary, this research provides a blueprint for clinicians and researchers to provide evidence for novel treatment of disease states with existing gene expression datasets. This preliminary work can be used within grant proposals to support the development of treatments through further testing in vivo, and in vitro. In addition, this methodology can be deployed quickly and at little cost other than the time of the investigator. Further steps in this research would be to facilitate data collection and analysis by consolidating the process within a single interface.

Limitations: Many genes play multiple roles during acute TBI reactions and cannot be squarely placed into specific pathways. Our gene analysis is not meant to present an exhaustive list of TBI relevant genes, but to highlight similarities in gene expression data across multiple curated TBI experiments. As a result, we recognize that some regulatory genes that may have evidence of strong contributions to the damaging effects of TBI may not be listed. All gene expression data used is limited to animal model TBI studies, and more research is needed to directly map these genes in human clinical studies. Additionally, gene pathway analysis and comparison among datasets yielded limited data for some genes. Not all genes could be identified or placed into gene pathways through the databases used, and it is difficult to differentiate in this context between "bad" and "good" inflammation. Inflammation is a natural response to injury and the way our body signals for repair. This inflammatory response when overwhelming can cause more damage, which seems to be the case for TBI. With TBI, treatment is more challenging because of the blood and brain barrier, making it difficult for many pharmacological therapies to cross.

We also recognize the limitations of our cheminformatic analysis. Perhaps one of the greatest limitations of the use of open-source resources is the overwhelming amount of information available, which can make it difficult to filter through and identify relevant data. For example, some molecule matches were part of indirect treatment studies by acting as a potent activator of immune system and inflammatory response. We ran ligands against all molecules for which data is accessible on PubChem. While PubChem does include findings from other chemical databases globally, many molecules may exist with similar properties as the ones mentioned that have yet to be recorded. Despite these limitations, we strove to present the most relevant information regarding relevant regulatory DEGs and the use of the listed matched molecules for TBI treatment while highlighting any notable exceptions.

While correlation-based methods are useful for identifying potential therapeutic targets, it is important to note that some ligands may inadvertently reduce the efficacy of pathways that are appropriately upregulated during the brain-injury response. For example, some pathways involved in inflammation or oxidative stress may play beneficial roles in the healing process, and suppressing these pathways could be counterproductive. Despite this limitation, the correlation approach remains valuable in identifying molecular leads that warrant further investigation in the context of therapeutic development. This method serves as an initial screening tool to pinpoint candidates for future experimental validation, allowing for a deeper exploration of their effects on both harmful and beneficial pathways.

While our study focused on secondary TBI, this approach could also be applied to other neurodegenerative conditions, such as Alzheimer's disease or stroke. By using similar cheminformatic and genomic methodologies, researchers could identify novel molecular leads targeting pathways related to oxidative stress, inflammation, and cell death—key factors in these diseases as well. This alternative application could expedite the discovery of therapeutic agents for conditions where current treatments are limited, similar to our findings for TBI.

Acknowledgments. This study was funded and supported by Dr. Jen Hayakawa and the Children's Hospital of Orange County Nursing and Informatics department.

Disclosure of Interests. The authors have no competing interests to declare that are relevant to the content of this article .

Appendix 1

See Table 5

Appendix 2

Appendix 3

See (Fig. 5)

Table 5. RCSB Ligand Identifier Information

RCSB Identifier	Compound Name	Ligand Type
CAD	Cacodylic Acid	Non-polymer
CDL	Cardiolipin	Non-polymer
EMJ	2,5-dihydroxy-3-undecylcyclohexa-2,5-diene-1,4-dione	Non-polymer
FMN	Flavin Mononucleotide	Non-polymer
GDE	Gallate	Non-polymer
HEA	Heme-A	Non-polymer
HEC	Heme-C	Non-polymer
HEM	Protoporphyrin IX Containing Fe	Non-polymer
INN	3,N(D,L-[2-(hydroxyamino-carbonyl)methyl]-4-methyl pentanoyl)L-3-(tert-butyl)glycyl-L-alanine	Peptide-like
KQV	[(2-{[(5S,8S,10aR)-3-acetyl-8-({(2S)-5-amino-1-[(diphenylmethyl)amino]-1,5-dioxopentan-2-yl}carbamoyl)-6-oxodecahydropyrrolo[1,2-a][1,5]diazocin-5-yl]carbamoyl}-1H-indol-5-yl)(difluoro)methyl]phosphonic acid	Non-polymer
K3Q	3,6-O-dimethyl-D-glucose	Non-polymer
MV0	7-acetyl-4-methoxy-1-benzofuran-3(2H)-one	Non-polymer
NAG	2-acetamido-2-deoxy-beta-D-glucopyranose	D-Saccharide, Beta Linking
NDP	NADPH dihydro-nicotinamide-adenine-dinucleotide phosphate	Non-polymer
PEE	1,2-dioleoyl-sn-glycero-3-phosphoethanolamine	Non-polymer
PLX	2-[hydroxy-[(2R)-3-[(1S)-1-hydroxyhexadecoxy]-2-[(1S)-1-hydroxyoctadecoxy]propoxy]phosphoryl]oxyethyl-trimethyl-azanium	Non-polymer
3PH	Phosphatidic Acid	Non-polymer
307	6,7-dimethyl-3-[[methyl-[2-[methyl-[[1-[3-(trifluoromethyl)phenyl]indol-3-yl]methyl]amino]ethyl]amino]methyl]chromen-4-one	Non-polymer
8Q1	S-dodecanoyl-4'-phosphopantetheine	Non-polymer

Table 6. List of the 95 small molecule matches found after PubChem's database of 22,000 + known molecules were run against 17 ligands identified from RCSB PDB.

PubChem Cid	Compound Name	Matched Ligand	Matched Gene/Protein
90467622	Iptacopan	307	TNF
44397540	2-(2-Methoxyphenyl)-1-(1-pentylindol-3-yl)etha-none	307	TNF
3686	Idebenone	EMJ	SERPINE1
129634336	Riboflavin thiamine	FMN	COX6C, NDUFB3, NDUFB9, NDUFV1
7048777	Riboflavine 5'-(dihydrogen phosphate), monoso-dium salt, dihydrate	FMN	COX6C, NDUFB3, NDUFB9, NDUFV1
493570	Riboflavin	FMN	COX6C, NDUFB3, NDUFB9, NDUFV1
4947	Propyl gallate	GDE	SERPINE1
370	Gallic Acid	GDE	SERPINE1
137528212	ME4fdg	K3Q	BCL2A1
71571511	Agar	K3Q	BCL2A1
44544736	Sgn-2FF	K3Q	BCL2A1
21627865	alpha-D-allofuranose	K3Q	BCL2A1
16666733	Pro-xylane	K3Q	BCL2A1
12303783	D-Paratose	K3Q	BCL2A1
12303780	L-Colitose	K3Q	BCL2A1
10975657	D-Ribose	K3Q	BCL2A1
10893439	Lauryl Glucoside	K3Q	BCL2A1
3232583	[18F]Fluorodeoxyglucose	K3Q	BCL2A1
2723872	D-Fructose	K3Q	BCL2A1
450503	Fludeoxyglucose F 18	K3Q	BCL2A1
445012	4-O-Acetyl-2,6-dideoxy-alpha-D-galacto-hexopy-ranose	K3Q	BCL2A1
444063	2,6-Dideoxy-beta-D-galactose	K3Q	BCL2A1
441036	D-Psicose	K3Q	BCL2A1
439764	beta-L-Arabinose	K3Q	BCL2A1
439507	D-Allose	K3Q	BCL2A1
439312	D-Tagatose	K3Q	BCL2A1
439268	D-Arabino-2-deoxyhexose	K3Q	BCL2A1
439195	L-Arabinose	K3Q	BCL2A1
369373	Dodecyl hexopyranoside	K3Q	BCL2A1
135191	D-Xylose	K3Q	BCL2A1
93321	Dodecyl beta-D-glucopyranoside	K3Q	BCL2A1
64960	1,5-Anhydro-D-glucitol	K3Q	BCL2A1
64689	beta-D-glucose	K3Q	BCL2A1
24310	beta-D-Fructopyranose	K3Q	BCL2A1
18950	D-Mannose	K3Q	BCL2A1
17106	L-Fucose	K3Q	BCL2A1
6036	D-Galactose	K3Q	BCL2A1
5793	D-Glucose	K3Q	BCL2A1
206	Hexose	K3Q	BCL2A1

(continued)

Table 6. (*continued*)

146395245	Kcy37T9rxu	KQV	STAT3
145343771	Unii-T5UX5skk2S	KQV	STAT3
15715157	8-Demethyleucalyptin	MV0	FOS
11611800	Benzoic acid, 3-((S)-(4-((4-acetyl-3-hydroxy-2-propylphenoxy)methyl)phenyl)hydroxymethyl)-	MV0	FOS
5318980	Icaritin	MV0	FOS
5281708	Daidzein	MV0	FOS
5280961	Genistein	MV0	FOS
5280863	Kaempferol	MV0	FOS
5280443	Apigenin	MV0	FOS
928465	Oxypeucedanin	MV0	FOS
667495	(2R)-5,7-dihydroxy-2-(4-hydroxyphenyl)-2,3-dihydro-4H-chromen-4-one	MV0	FOS
480764	8-Prenylnaringenin	MV0	FOS
442614	(+)-Usnic acid	MV0	FOS
441140	Griseofulvin	MV0	FOS
439246	Naringenin	MV0	FOS
155094	6-Prenylnaringenin	MV0	FOS
114829	Liquiritigenin	MV0	FOS
68081	Isoimperatorin	MV0	FOS
68079	Isopimpinellin	MV0	FOS
68071	Pinocembrin	MV0	FOS
11092	Paeonol	MV0	FOS
10658	Angelicin	MV0	FOS
10212	Pentosalen	MV0	FOS
8569	Dioxybenzone	MV0	FOS
6758	Rotenone	MV0	FOS
6199	Psoralen	MV0	FOS
5646	Usnic acid	MV0	FOS
5585	Trioxsalen	MV0	FOS
4825	Pimpinellin	MV0	FOS
4632	Oxybenzone	MV0	FOS
4114	Methoxsalen	MV0	FOS
3512	Gris-PEG	MV0	FOS
2355	Bergapten	MV0	FOS
932	5,7-Dihydroxy-2-(4-hydroxyphenyl)chroman-4-one	MV0	FOS
138403271	1-methyl-1-nitroso-3-[(3R,4R,5S)-2,4,5-trihydroxy-6-(hydroxymethyl)oxan-3-yl]urea	NAG	ICAM, IL6, IL1B, TLR2, IL1R2
137332080	2-deoxy-2-[(difluoroacetyl)amino]-alpha-D-galactopyranose	NAG	ICAM, IL6, IL1B, TLR2, IL1R2
134695375	1-methyl-1-nitroso-3-[(2S,3R,4R)-2,4,5-trihydroxy-6-(hydroxymethyl)oxan-3-yl]urea	NAG	ICAM, IL6, IL1B, TLR2, IL1R2
45357367	Streptozotocin (streptozocin)	NAG	ICAM, IL6, IL1B, TLR2, IL1R2

(*continued*)

Table 6. (*continued*)

7067772	2-Deoxy-2-(3-methyl-3-nitrosoureido)-D-gluco-pyranose	NAG	ICAM, IL6, IL1B, TLR2, IL1R2
6713972	1-methyl-1-nitroso-3-[(2S,4S,5S)-2,4,5-trihy-droxy-6-(hydroxymethyl)oxan-3-yl]urea	NAG	ICAM, IL6, IL1B, TLR2, IL1R2
6420074	Streptozocin (streptozotocin)	NAG	ICAM, IL6, IL1B, TLR2, IL1R2
2733335	2-deoxy-2-[[(methylnitrosoamino)car-bonyl]amino]-D-glucose	NAG	ICAM, IL6, IL1B, TLR2, IL1R2
441477	beta-D-Glucosamine	NAG	ICAM, IL6, IL1B, TLR2, IL1R2
439281	N-Acetyl-D-Mannosamine	NAG	ICAM, IL6, IL1B, TLR2, IL1R2
439213	D-Glucosamine	NAG	ICAM, IL6, IL1B, TLR2, IL1R2
439174	N-Acetyl-D-Glucosamine	NAG	ICAM, IL6, IL1B, TLR2, IL1R2
29327	Streptozocin	NAG	ICAM, IL6, IL1B, TLR2, IL1R2
24139	N-ACETYL-beta-D-GLUCOSAMINE	NAG	ICAM, IL6, IL1B, TLR2, IL1R2
5300	D-Glucose, 2-deoxy-2-[[(methylnitrosoamino)-carbonyl]amino]-	NAG	ICAM, IL6, IL1B, TLR2, IL1R2
9802422	(2r,4ar,6r,7r,7as)-6-(6-Amino-8-Bromo-9h-Purin-9-Yl)tetrahydro-4h-Furo[3,2-D][1,3,2]dioxaphos-phinine-2,7-Diol 2-Sulfide	NDP	COX6C, NDUFB3, NDUFB9, NDUFV1
6858240	Sp-Camps	NDP	COX6C, NDUFB3, NDUFB9, NDUFV1
100299	Tocladesine	NDP	COX6C, NDUFB3, NDUFB9, NDUFV1
60961	Adenosine	NDP	COX6C, NDUFB3, NDUFB9, NDUFV1
24405	Riboprine	NDP	COX6C, NDUFB3, NDUFB9, NDUFV1
21704	Vidarabine	NDP	COX6C, NDUFB3, NDUFB9, NDUFV1
6076	Adenosine cyclic phosphate	NDP	COX6C, NDUFB3, NDUFB9, NDUFV1

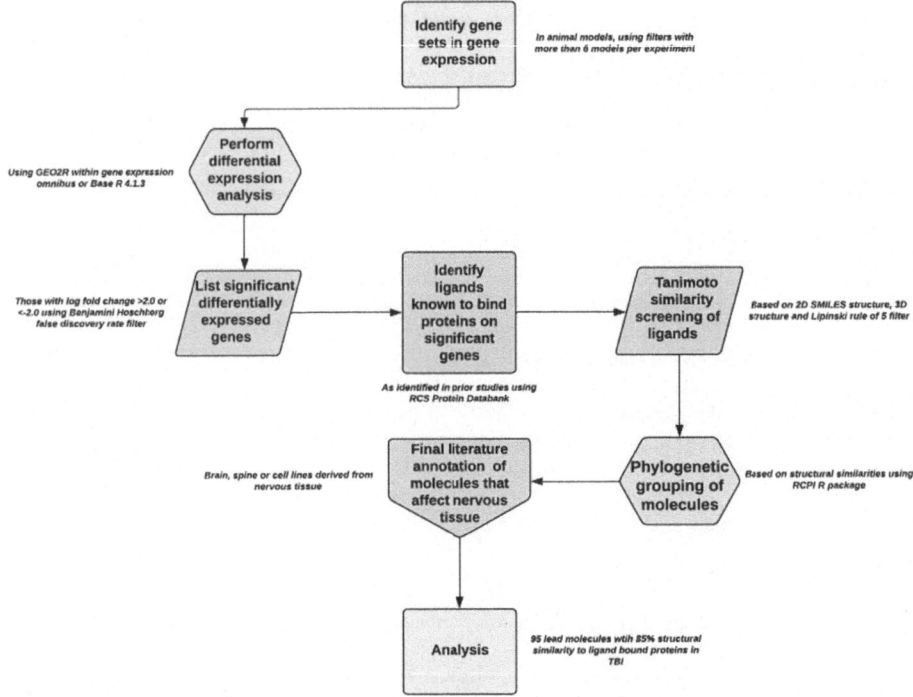

Fig. 5. Sequence of Methodology

References

1. Langlois, J.A., Rutland-Brown, W., Wald, M.M.: The epidemiology and impact of traumatic brain injury: a brief overview. J. Head Trauma Rehabil. **21**(5), 375–378 (2006)
2. Taylor, C.A., Bell, J.M., Breiding, M.J., Xu, L.: Traumatic brain injury-related emergency department visits, hospitalizations, and deaths—United States, 2007 and 2013. MMWR Surveill. Summ. **66**(9), 1–16 (2017). https://doi.org/10.15585/mmwr.ss6609a1
3. Harrison-Felix, C., et al.: Mortality after surviving traumatic brain injury: risks based on age groups. J. Head Trauma Rehabilit. **27**(6), E45–E56 (2012)
4. McKee, A.C., Robinson, M.E.: Military-related traumatic brain injury and neurodegeneration. Alzheimers Dement. **10**(3 Suppl), S242–S253 (2014). https://doi.org/10.1016/j.jalz.2014.04.003, PMID:24924675; PMCID:PMC4255273
5. Popernack, M.L., Gray, N., Reuter-Rice, K.: Moderate-to-severe traumatic brain injury in children: complications and rehabilitation strategies. J. Pediatr. Health Care **29**(3), e1–e7 (2015)
6. Sahler, C.S., Greenwald, B.D.: Traumatic brain injury in sports: a review. Rehabil. Res. Pract. **2012**, 659652 (2012). https://doi.org/10.1155/2012/659652. Epub 2012 Jul 9. PMID: 22848836; PMCID: PMC3400421
7. Shah, S., Kimberly, W. T.: Today's approach to treating brain swelling in the neuro intensive care unit. Seminars Neurol. **36**(06), 502–507 (2016). https://doi.org/10.1055/s-0036-1592109
8. Needham, E.J., Helmy, A., Zanier, E.R., Jones, J.L., Coles, A.J., Menon, D.K.: The immunological response to traumatic brain injury. J. Neuroimmunol. **332**, 112–125 (2019)

9. Schomberg, J.: Identification of targetable pathways in oral cancer patients via random forest and chemical informatics. Cancer Inform. **18**, 1176935119889911 (2019). https://doi.org/10.1177/1176935119889911

10. Petersen, A., Soderstrom, M., Saha, B., Sharma, P.: Animal models of traumatic brain injury: a review of pathophysiology to biomarkers and treatments. Exp. Brain Res. **239**, 2939–2950 (2021)

11. Shojo, H., Kaneko, Y., Mabuchi, T., Kibayashi, K., Adachi, N., Borlongan, C.V.: Genetic and histo-logic evidence implicates role of inflammation in traumatic brain injury-induced apoptosis in the rat cerebral cortex following moderate fluid percussion injury. Neuroscience **171**(4), 1273–1282 (2010). https://doi.org/10.1016/j.neuroscience.2010.10.018. Epub 2010 Oct 13 PMID: 20950674

12. Shojo, H., Borlongan, C.V., Mabuchi, T.: Genetic and histological alterations reveal key role of prostaglandin synthase and cyclooxygenase 1 and 2 in traumatic brain injury-induced neu-roinflammation in the cerebral cortex of rats exposed to moderate fluid percussion injury. Cell Transplant. **26**(7), 1301–1313 (2017). https://doi.org/10.1177/0963689717715169. PMID:28933223; PMCID:PMC5657737

13. Lipponen, A., Paananen, J., Puhakka, N., Pitkänen, A.: Analysis of post-traumatic brain injury gene expression signature reveals tubulins, Nfe2l2, Nfkb, Cd44, and S100a4 as treatment targets. Sci. Rep. **17**(6), 31570 (2016). https://doi.org/10.1038/srep31570 . PMID:27530814; PMCID:PMC4987651

14. White, T.E., Ford, G.D., Surles-Zeigler, M.C., Gates, A.S., et al.: Gene expression patterns following unilateral traumatic brain injury reveals a local pro-inflammatory and remote anti-inflammatory response. BMC Genomics **25**(14), 282 (2013). PMID: 23617241

15. Ng, J.M., Chen, M.J., Leung, J.Y., Peng, Z.F., et al.: Transcriptional insights on the regenerative mechanics of axotomized neurons in vitro. J. Cell. Mol. Med. **16**(4), 789–811 (2012). PMID: 21711447

16. Paban, V., et al.: Changes in gene expression following experimental traumatic brain injury; similarities with changes following stroke and depression. J. Trans. Sci. **2**(6): 330–339 (2016)

17. Paban, V., et al.: Changes in gene expression following experimental traumatic brain injury; similarities with changes following stroke and depression. J. Trans. Sci. **2**(6), 330–339 (2016)

18. Love, M.I., Huber, W., Anders, S.: Moderated estimation of fold change and dispersion for RNA-seq data with DESeq2. Genome Biol. **15**(12), 550 (2014). https://doi.org/10.1186/s13059-014-0550-8

19. Boone, D.R., Weisz, H.A., Willey, H.E., Torres, K.E.O., et al.: Traumatic brain injury induces long-lasting changes in immune and regenerative signaling. PLoS ONE **14**(4), e0214741 (2019). PMID: 30943276

20. Edgar, R., Domrachev, M., Lash, A.E.: Gene Expression Omnibus: NCBI gene expression and hybridization array data repository. Nucleic Acids Res. **30**(1), 207–210 (2002)

21. Fabregat, A., Sidiropoulos, K., Viteri, G., et al.: Reactome pathway analysis: a high-performance in-memory approach. BMC Bioinform **18**, 142 (2017). https://doi.org/10.1186/s12859-017-1559-2

22. Szklarczyk, D.: The STRING database in 2023: protein–protein association networks and functional enrichment analyses for any sequenced genome of interest

23. Berman, H.M., et al.: The protein data bank. Nucleic Acids Res. **28**, 235–242 (2000). https://doi.org/10.1093/nar/28.1.235. https://www.rcsb.org/

24. Chung, NC., Miasojedow, B., Startek, M., Gambin A.: Jaccard/Tanimoto similarity test and estimation methods for biological presence-absence data. BMC Bioinform. **20** (Suppl15), 644 (2019). arXiv:1903.11372. https://doi.org/10.1186/s12859-019-3118-5. PMC 6929325. PMID 31874610

25. Seo, M., Shin, H.K., Myung, Y., et al.: Development of natural compound molecular finger-print (NC-MFP) with the dictionary of natural products (DNP) for natural product-based drug development. J. Cheminform. **12**, 6 (2020). https://doi.org/10.1186/s13321-020-0410-3

26. He, W., Hu, Z., Zhong, Y., Wu, C., Li, J.: The potential of NLRP3 inflammasome as a therapeutic target in neurological diseases. Mol. Neurobiol. **60**(5), 2520–2538 (2023). https://doi.org/10.1007/s12035-023-03229-7

27. Luo, T., Jia, X., Feng, W., et al.: Bergapten inhibits NLRP3 inflammasome activation and pyroptosis via promoting mitophagy. Acta Pharmacol. Sin. **44**, 1867–1878 (2023). https://doi.org/10.1038/s41401-023-01094-7

28. Wang, T., et al.: Pinocembrin suppresses oxidized low-density lipoprotein-triggered NLRP3 inflammasome/GSDMD-mediated endothelial cell pyroptosis through an Nrf2-dependent signaling pathway. Sci. Rep. **12**(1) (2022). https://doi.org/10.1038/s41598-022-18297-3

29. Peng, J., et al.: Idebenone attenuates cerebral inflammatory injury in ischemia and reperfusion via dampening NLRP3 inflammasome activity. Mol. Immunol. **123**, 74–87 (2020). https://doi.org/10.1016/j.molimm.2020.04.013

30. Vijayalakshmi, P., Indu, S., Ireen, C., Manjunathan, R., Rajalakshmi, M.: Octyl gallate and gallic acid isolated from terminalia bellirica circumvent breast cancer progression by enhancing the intrinsic apoptotic signaling pathway and elevating the levels of anti-oxidant enzymes. Appl. Biochem. Biotechnol. (2023). https://doi.org/10.1007/s12010-023-04450-9. Advance online publication

31. Chen, L., et al.: A comprehensive review of its botany, traditional uses, phytochemistry, pharmacology, toxicology, quality control and pharmacokinetics. Chin. Med. **18**(1), 4 (2023). https://doi.org/10.1186/s13020-022-00704-6

32. Engin, B., Oguz, O.: Evaluation of time-dependent response to psoralen plus UVA (PUVA) treatment with topical 8-methoxypsoralen (8-MOP) gel in palmoplantar dermatoses. Int. J. Dermatol. **44**(4), 337–339 (2005)

33. Hui, Y., Zhao, H., Shi, L., et al.: Traumatic brain injury-mediated neuroinflammation and neurological deficits are improved by 8-Methoxypsoralen through modulating PPARγ/NF-κB pathway. Neurochem. Res. **48**, 625–640 (2023). https://doi.org/10.1007/s11064-022-03788-6

34. Cai, L., Zeng, R., Huang, Q., Liu, X., Cao, Z., Guo, Q.: Paeonol inhibits chronic constriction injury-induced astrocytic activation and neuroinflammation in rats via the HDAC/miR-15a pathway. Drug Dev. Res. **83**(8), 1758–1765 (2022). https://doi.org/10.1002/ddr.21993

35. Viswanatha, G.L., Shylaja, H., Moolemath, Y.: The beneficial role of Naringin- a citrus bioflavonoid, against oxidative stress-induced neurobehavioral disorders and cognitive dysfunction in rodents: a systematic review and meta-analysis. Biomed. Pharmacotherapy **94**, 909–929 (2017). https://doi.org/10.1016/j.biopha.2017.07.072

36. Paramanik, V., Kurrey, K., Singh, P., et al.: Roles of genistein in learning and memory during aging and neurological disorders. Biogerontology **24**, 329–346 (2023). https://doi.org/10.1007/s10522-023-10020-7

37. Soltani, Z., Khaksari, M., Jafari, E., Iranpour, M., Shahrokhi, N.: Is genistein neu-roprotective in traumatic brain injury? Physiol. Behav. **152**(Pt A), 26–31 (2015). https://doi.org/10.1016/j.physbeh.2015.08.037

38. Zhang, M., et al.: Biomimetic remodeling of microglial riboflavin metabolism ame-liorates cognitive impairment by modulating neuroinflammation. Adv. Sci. (Weinheim, Baden-Wurttemberg, Germany) **10**(12), e2300180 (2023). https://doi.org/10.1002/advs.202300180

39. Tang, Y.L., Fang, L.J., Zhong, L.Y., Jiang, J., Dong, X.Y., Feng, Z.: Hub genes and key pathways of traumatic brain injury: bioinformatics analysis and: in vivo: valida-tion. Neural Regen. Res. **15**(12), 2262–2269 (2020)

40. Wang, X., et al.: Clarifying the mechanism of apigenin against blood-brain barrier disruption in ischemic stroke using systems pharmacology. Mol. Diversity (2023). https://doi.org/10.1007/s11030-023-10607-9. Advance online publication
41. Kremer, M., Glennerster, R.: Strong medicine: creating incentives for pharmaceuti-cal research on neglected diseases. Princeton University Press (2004)

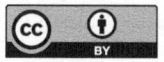

Investigating the Need for Personalized Assessment: An Example from Thyroid Function Tests

Ricardo A. Aguilar[1]($\boxtimes$) (iD), Louis Ehwerhemuepha[1] (iD), and Terence Sanger[1,2] (iD)

[1] Children's Hospital of Orange County, Orange, CA 92868, USA
{Ricardo.Aguilar,LEhwerhemuepha,Terence.Sanger}@choc.org
[2] School of Medicine, University of California, Irvine, CA 92617, USA

Abstract. Using population-wide thresholds assumes normal variation in thyroid hormone levels is the same across individuals which may leave patients (with varying medical histories) undiagnosed and untreated. This analysis aims to assess whether patient-specific thresholds for thyroid hormone laboratory tests are justifiable within a heterogeneous pediatric population.

The study data, obtained from Cerner Real-World Data, consists of observations from January 2016 to December 2019 of pediatric patients with at least two laboratory records for thyrotropin (TSH), free thyroxine (T4), total T4, or free triiodothyronine (T3) tests.

Linear mixed models were built to estimate patient-specific ranges and variance partition coefficients (VPCs) while controlling for various patient characteristics.

Inclusion criteria resulted in 97,195 observations across 31,170 patients for TSH; 229,523 observations across 68,396 patients for free T4; 32,346 observations across 10,201 patients for total T4; and 6,994 observations across 2,557 patients for free T3.

Decision-making inconsistencies occurred for 15.1% of TSH, 29.5% of free T4, 18.4% of total T4, and 17.9% of free T3 values. The average VPC estimates suggest inter-subject variation explains 21% (95% CI: 0.21–0.22), 28% (95% CI: 0.27–0.29), 41% (95% CI: 0.39–0.43), and 26% (95% CI: 0.23–0.29) of total variation in TSH, free T4, total T4, and free T3, respectively.

Although commonly used, population ranges may lead to diagnostic errors. Inconsistencies were found in at least 15% of thyroid hormone laboratory values and inter-subject variation explains at least 20% of total variation in these thyroid hormone tests. This study's results suggest patient-specific ranges are justifiable and may reduce diagnostic errors.

Keywords: Pediatrics · Thyroid Tests · Individualized Medicine

1 Introduction

Use of population-wide thresholds assumes that normal variation in thyroid hormone levels is the same across individuals. Thyroid hormone levels are measured and compared to agreed-upon thresholds to diagnose thyroid conditions, such as hypothyroidism or

© The Author(s) 2025
L. Ehwerhemuepha et al. (Eds.): IPLDSC 2024, CCIS 2386, pp. 72–80, 2025.
https://doi.org/10.1007/978-3-031-88346-0_5

hyperthyroidism [1]. The push for individualized medicine [2–4] has created a need to reevaluate the use of population-wide (and sometimes age-specific) [1, 5] thresholds. Even in those exhibiting symptoms, screening for thyroid conditions using population thresholds can have a low yield of positive results [6] which may leave some patients undiagnosed and, consequently, untreated. This analysis aims to assess whether patient-specific thresholds are justified for laboratory measures of thyroid hormone production within a large, heterogenous, and pediatric patient population.

2 Methods

The study data were obtained from Cerner Real-World Data, a large multicenter electronic health records database, under the Children's Hospital of Orange County Institutional Review Board (IRB #2008107). The data consists of observations from January 2016 to December 2019 where patients are at most 18 years old and have at least two laboratory records for thyrotropin (TSH) mIU/L, free thyroxine (T4) ng/dl, total T4 µg/dL, or free triiodothyronine (T3) pg/mL blood tests. Using diagnosis and procedure codes as described by Feudtner et al., this study adopted the definitions for pediatric complex chronic condition (CCC) classifications [7].

A linear mixed model for each thyroid hormone laboratory measure (as the outcome) was built with random intercepts for each patient and health system and quadratic random slope terms for age for each patient while controlling for demographics, CCCs, prior year thyroid medication history, and thyroid condition history. These models were used to estimate patient-specific ranges through prediction intervals and variance partition coefficients (VPCs). In this study, a VPC of 0.20 can be interpreted as, "20% of the total variance is explained by differences between patients." Inconsistencies (decisions based on patient and population range not in agreement) were investigated using a simple random sample of individual laboratory measures (i.e. a random sample where multiple laboratory measures from the same patient are possible). The random sample was limited to 1,000 observations because accurate prediction intervals are computationally intensive for linear mixed models. This is due to the necessity of accounting for variation in the random effects in addition to the variation in the fixed effects and residuals. Statistical analyses were conducted using R version 4.1.2 and the rptR package [8].

3 Results

Inclusion criteria resulted in 97,195 observations across 31,170 patients for TSH; 229,523 observations across 68,396 patients for free T4; 32,346 observations across 10,201 patients for total T4; and 6,994 observations across 2,557 patients for free T3. Summary statistics for patient characteristics are contained in Table 1.

Inconsistencies occurred for 15.1% of TSH, 29.5% of free T4, 18.4% of total T4, and 17.9% of free T3 values (Table 2). The average VPC estimates in Table 3 suggest inter-subject variation explains 21% (95% CI: 0.21–0.22), 28% (95% CI: 0.27–0.29), 41% (95% CI: 0.39–0.43), and 26% (95% CI: 0.23–0.29) of total variation in TSH, free T4, total T4, and free T3, respectively.

Table 1. Summary statistics by thyroid laboratory test.

Variable	TSH (mIU/L), mean (sd), n (%)	Free T4 (ng/dL), mean (sd), n (%)	Total T4 (µg/dL), mean (sd), n (%)	Free T3 (pg/mL), mean (sd), n (%)
Outcomes[1]				
Laboratory Values	2.86 (2.79)	1.22 (0.32)	8.48 (3.01)	4.07 (2.10)
Demographics				
Age1	11.17 (5.25)	10.40 (5.50)	10.46 (5.24)	12.26 (4.93)
Gender2				
Female	18,033 (57.85)	39,048 (57.09)	5,765 (56.51)	1,588 (62.10)
Male	13,048 (41.86)	29,171 (42.65)	4,336 (42.51)	943 (36.88)
Unknown/Other	89 (0.29)	177 (0.26)	100 (0.98)	26 (1.02)
Race/Ethnicity2				
American Indian or Alaska Native	154 (0.49)	465 (0.68)	48 (0.47)	24 (0.94)
Asian	813 (2.61)	1,888 (2.76)	275 (2.70)	100 (3.91)
Black or African American	3,433 (11.01)	7,079 (10.35)	436 (4.27)	187 (7.31)
Hispanic or Latino	6,139 (19.70)	13,655 (19.96)	3,106 (30.45)	389 (15.21)
Native Hawaiian or Other Pacific Islander	33 (0.11)	82 (0.12)	22 (0.22)	1 (0.04)
Other or Unknown	5,985 (19.20)	8,881 (12.98)	2,338 (22.92)	529 (20.69)
White	14,613 (46.88)	36,346 (53.14)	3,976 (38.98)	1,327 (51.9)
Complex Chronic Conditions[2]				
Cardiovascular				
No	29,704 (93.41)	64,020 (90.62)	9,656 (93.13)	2,417 (93.39)
Yes	2,097 (6.59)	6,625 (9.38)	712 (6.87)	171 (6.61)
Congenital/Genetic				
No	27,863 (86.65)	60,505 (84.36)	9,177 (87.11)	2,373 (91.34)
Yes	4,291 (13.35)	11,219 (15.64)	1,358 (12.89)	225 (8.66)

(continued)

Table 1. (*continued*)

Variable	TSH (mIU/L), mean (sd), n (%)	Free T4 (ng/dL), mean (sd), n (%)	Total T4 (µg/dL), mean (sd), n (%)	Free T3 (pg/mL), mean (sd), n (%)
Gastrointestinal				
No	30,393 (96.36)	66,227 (95.11)	9,908 (96.08)	2,502 (97.47)
Yes	1,149 (3.64)	3,408 (4.89)	404 (3.92)	65 (2.53)
Hematologic/Immunologic				
No	30,280 (95.94)	65,973 (94.60)	9,925 (96.24)	2,440 (94.35)
Yes	1,281 (4.06)	3,767 (5.40)	388 (3.76)	146 (5.65)
Metabolic				
No	27,787 (82.51)	59,933 (80.67)	9,002 (80.92)	2,316 (87.13)
Yes	5,890 (17.49)	14,362 (19.33)	2,123 (19.08)	342 (12.87)
Neonatology/Prematurity				
No	30,471 (97.51)	66,199 (96.36)	9,929 (97.08)	2,514 (98.24)
Yes	779 (2.49)	2,504 (3.64)	299 (2.92)	45 (1.76)
Neoplasms				
No	30,276 (96.53)	65,735 (95.18)	9,934 (96.83)	2,469 (96.11)
Yes	1,088 (3.47)	3,329 (4.82)	325 (3.17)	100 (3.89)
Neurologic				
No	29,640 (93.24)	64,220 (91.11)	9,664 (93.16)	2,445 (94.62)
Yes	2,150 (6.76)	6,267 (8.89)	710 (6.84)	139 (5.38)
Devices/Implants/Transplants				
No	31,054 (99.22)	68,029 (98.78)	10,136 (98.82)	2,546 (99.34)
Yes	244 (0.78)	839 (1.22)	121 (1.18)	17 (0.66)
Renal/Urologic				
No	30,711 (97.78)	67,139 (97.19)	10,024 (97.60)	2,524 (98.36)

(*continued*)

Table 1. (*continued*)

Variable	TSH (mIU/L), mean (sd), n (%)	Free T4 (ng/dL), mean (sd), n (%)	Total T4 (µg/dL), mean (sd), n (%)	Free T3 (pg/mL), mean (sd), n (%)
Yes	698 (2.22)	1,940 (2.81)	246 (2.40)	42 (1.64)
Respiratory				
No	30,713 (98.11)	66,933 (96.95)	9,977 (97.21)	2,520 (98.25)
Yes	592 (1.89)	2,107 (3.05)	286 (2.79)	45 (1.75)
Thyroid Medications[1]				
Levothyroxine				
No	73,506 (75.63)	158,996 (69.27)	23,031 (71.20)	5,933 (84.83)
Yes	23,689 (24.37)	70,527 (30.73)	9,315 (28.80)	1,061 (15.17)
Liothyronine				
No	96,874 (99.67)	228,956 (99.75)	32,314 (99.90)	6,873 (98.27)
Yes	321 (0.33)	567 (0.25)	32 (0.10)	121 (1.73)
Thyroid Desiccated				
No	97,126 (99.93)	229,431 (99.96)	32,344 (99.99)	6,944 (99.29)
Yes	69 (0.07)	92 (0.04)	2 (0.01)	50 (0.71)
Thyrotropin Alfa				
No	97,183 (99.99)	229,491 (99.99)	32,337 (99.97)	6,993 (99.99)
Yes	12 (0.01)	32 (0.01)	9 (0.03)	1 (0.01)
Methimazole				
No	94,176 (96.89)	222,803 (97.07)	30,831 (95.32)	6,372 (91.11)
Yes	3,019 (3.11)	6,720 (2.93)	1,515 (4.68)	622 (8.89)
Propylthiouracil				
No	97,183 (99.99)	229,503 (99.99)	32,339 (99.98)	6,986 (99.89)
Yes	12 (0.01)	20 (0.01)	7 (0.02)	8 (0.11)
Thyroid Conditions[1]				

(*continued*)

Table 1. (*continued*)

Variable	TSH (mIU/L), mean (sd), n (%)	Free T4 (ng/dL), mean (sd), n (%)	Total T4 (µg/dL), mean (sd), n (%)	Free T3 (pg/mL), mean (sd), n (%)
Hashimoto's Thyroiditis				
No	90,239 (92.84)	206,123 (89.80)	28,826 (89.12)	6,566 (93.88)
Yes	6,956 (7.16)	23,400 (10.20)	3,520 (10.88)	428 (6.12)
Hyperthyroidism				
No	92,392 (95.06)	217,401 (94.72)	29,448 (91.04)	5,951 (85.09)
Yes	4,803 (4.94)	12,122 (5.28)	2,898 (8.96)	1,043 (14.91)
Hypothyroidism				
No	69,443 (71.45)	146,312 (63.75)	19,137 (59.16)	5,229 (74.76)
Yes	27,752 (28.55)	83,211 (36.25)	13,209 (40.84)	1,765 (25.24)
Other Thyroid Disorder				
No	91,067 (93.70)	211,407 (92.11)	28,585 (88.37)	6,194 (88.56)
Yes	6,128 (6.30)	18,116 (7.89)	3,761 (11.63)	800 (11.44)
Other Thyroiditis				
No	96,678 (99.47)	227,276 (99.02)	31,995 (98.91)	6,915 (98.87)
Yes	517 (0.53)	2,247 (0.98)	351 (1.09)	79 (1.13)

[1] Any characteristic or group of characteristics whose summary statistics are at the laboratory measure (observation) level. [2] Gender, race and ethnicity, and complex chronic condition summary statistics are at the patient level. It should be noted that complex chronic condition counts may have repeated cases for a patient if their status changed between observations. Any binary variables with fewer than 10 observations recorded as "Yes" for a given laboratory measure were excluded from that model, due to statistical separability issues, but were kept in the summary statistics table to show their distributions for models in which there were no such issues

4 Discussion

Although commonly used, population ranges may lead to diagnostic errors. Inconsistencies were found in at least 15% of thyroid hormone laboratory values. Of the 1,000 randomly sampled laboratory measures, 20.0% of TSH, 37.8% of free T4, 33.3% of total T4, and 75.0% of free T3 values within their population range [1, 5] and outside of their estimated patient-specific range were not on medications. This finding suggests that

Table 2. Counts for population and patient range status from sample of 1,000 laboratory measures.

TSH	Population Range Normal	Population Range Abnormal
Patient Range Normal	797	141
Patient Range Abnormal	10	52

Of the 10 measures within their population normal range and outside of their patient-specific range, 20.0% were not on medication.

Free T4	Population Range Normal	Population Range Abnormal
Patient Range Normal	668	258
Patient Range Abnormal	37	37

Of the 37 measures within their population normal range and outside of their patient-specific range, 37.8% were not on medication.

Total T4	Population Range Normal	Population Range Abnormal
Patient Range Normal	769	160
Patient Range Abnormal	24	47

Of the 24 measures within their population normal range and outside of their patient-specific range, 33.3% were not on medication.

Free T3	Population Range Normal	Population Range Abnormal
Patient Range Normal	764	163
Patient Range Abnormal	16	57

Of the 16 measures within their population normal range and outside of their patient-specific range, 75.0% were not on medication.

adherence to population-based ranges may lead to undertreatment in a significant number of hypo- and hyperthyroidism patients. Additionally, the estimated average VPCs suggest that differences across patients' average thyroid hormone levels explain greater than 20% of total variation. This study's results suggest that patient-specific ranges are justifiable and may be necessary in reducing diagnostic errors.

The models in this study include fixed effects for whether patients had a recorded diagnosis for each of the thyroid conditions listed in Table 1. and whether they received any corresponding medications within a year prior to when the thyroid hormone laboratory measures were obtained. Thus, the estimated patient-specific ranges and VPCs adjust for the temporal relationships between diagnosis, treatment, and laboratory measures across a patient's multiple encounters. Potential distributional violations were examined by applying square root, fourth root, and logarithmic transformations to the outcomes; results were consistent with their non-transformed counterparts.

In practice, health systems can build models for their respective patient populations by using their own electronic health records. For new laboratory measures, patients' data can be automatically retrieved and run through the model to estimate patient-specific ranges in real-time. The estimated ranges can then be displayed and used by clinicians for screening or diagnostic purposes. Further research to quantify such ranges using reinforcement learning (that can more precisely estimate a patient's healthy range) in conjunction with clinical expertise is needed.

Table 3. Sample sizes and linear mixed modeling results.

	TSH (mIU/L)	Free T4 (ng/dL)	Total T4 (µg/dL)	Free T3 (pg/mL)
Sample Sizes				
Total Sample Size	97,195	229,523	32,346	6,994
Number of Patients	31,170	68,396	10,201	2,557
VPC and Variance Components of Mixed Effects Modelsa				
VPC	0.21 (0.21, 0.22)	0.28 (0.27, 0.29)	0.41 (0.39, 0.43)	0.26 (0.23, 0.29)
Inter-Subject Variance	1.65 (1.58, 1.71)	0.03 (0.03, 0.03)	4.07 (3.91, 4.23)	1.02 (0.91, 1.15)
Health System Variance	0.11 (0.06, 0.18)	0.01 (0.01, 0.02)	0.66 (0.37, 1.03)	0.26 (0.14, 0.41)
Fixed Effects Variance	0.58 (0.55, 0.63)	0.01 (0.01, 0.01)	1.57 (1.43, 1.71)	0.56 (0.50, 0.68)
Intra-Subject Variance	5.41 (5.35, 5.46)	0.05 (0.05, 0.05)	3.56 (3.49, 3.63)	2.15 (2.05, 2.23)

[a]When most groups have only two or three observations, linear mixed models produce adjusted and robust but conservative estimates (due to shrinkage) of group-level variance components and, consequently, VPCs. All confidence intervals shown are parametric bootstrap confidence intervals. TSH, thyrotropin; T4, thyroxine; T3, triiodothyronine; VPC, variance partition coefficient

Acknowledgments. Thank you to Dr. Lois Sayrs for her review of the manuscript and feedback.

Disclosure of Interests. The authors have no competing interests to declare that are relevant to the content of this article.

References

1. Elmlinger, M.W., Kühnel, W., Lambrecht, H.-G., Ranke, M.B.: Reference intervals from birth to adulthood for Serum Thyroxine (T4), Triiodothyronine (T3), free T3, free T4, Thyroxine Binding Globulin (TBG) and Thyrotropin (TSH). Clin. Chem. Lab. Med. **39**, 973–979 (2001). https://doi.org/10.1515/CCLM.2001.158
2. Topol, E.J.: Individualized medicine from Prewomb to tomb. Cell **157**, 241–253 (2014). https://doi.org/10.1016/j.cell.2014.02.012
3. Johnson, K.B., et al.: Precision medicine, ai, and the future of personalized health care. Clin Transl Sci. **14**, 86–93 (2021). https://doi.org/10.1111/cts.12884
4. Ho, D., et al.: Enabling technologies for personalized and precision medicine. Trends Biotechnol. **38**, 497–518 (2020). https://doi.org/10.1016/j.tibtech.2019.12.021
5. Lem, A.J., et al.: Serum thyroid hormone levels in healthy children from birth to adulthood and in short children born small for gestational age. J. Clin. Endocrinol. Metab. **97**, 3170–3178 (2012). https://doi.org/10.1210/jc.2012-1759

6. Reinehr, T., Hinney, A., de Sousa, G., Austrup, F., Hebebrand, J., Andler, W.: Definable somatic disorders in overweight children and adolescents. J. Pediatr. **150**, 618-622.e5 (2007). https://doi.org/10.1016/j.jpeds.2007.01.042
7. Feudtner, C., Feinstein, J.A., Zhong, W., Hall, M., Dai, D.: Pediatric complex chronic conditions classification system version 2: updated for ICD-10 and complex medical technology dependence and transplantation. BMC Pediatr. **14** (2014). https://doi.org/10.1186/1471-2431-14-199
8. Stoffel, M.A., Nakagawa, S., Schielzeth, H.: RptR: Repeatability estimation and variance decomposition by generalized linear mixed-effects models. Methods Ecol. Evol.Evol. **8**, 1639–1644 (2017). https://doi.org/10.1111/2041-210X.12797

Correction to: Identification of Molecular Leads for Treatment of Secondary TBI via Analysis of Gene Expression in Models of Traumatic Brain Injury in Combination with Two-Dimensional and Three-Dimensional Drug Library Analysis

Sarah Randall⬤, Andreina Giron⬤, Zoe Flyer⬤, Alice Martino⬤, and John Schomberg⬤

Correction to:
Chapter 4 in: L. Ehwerhemuepha et al. (Eds.): *Pediatric and Lifespan Data Science*, CCIS 2386, https://doi.org/10.1007/978-3-031-88346-0_4

In the originally published version of chapter 4, the order of authors had been rendered incorrectly. This has been corrected.

The updated version of this chapter can be found at
https://doi.org/10.1007/978-3-031-88346-0_4

© The Author(s) 2025
L. Ehwerhemuepha et al. (Eds.): IPLDSC 2024, CCIS 2386, p. C1, 2025.
https://doi.org/10.1007/978-3-031-88346-0_6

Machine Learning Models for Prediction of Sepsis in Pediatric Patients

Jacqueline Lee[1,2], Aline Rohloff[1(✉)], and Robert Kelly[1,2]

[1] Children's Hospital of Orange County, Orange, CA 92868, USA
{jacqueline.lee, arohloff}@choc.org
[2] University of California Irvine, Irvine, CA 92697, USA

Abstract. This report summarizes a panel from the Pediatric and Lifespan Data Science Conference entitled "Sepsis: Current Practices and Opportunities for Artificial Intelligence (AI) Applications." Sepsis is a progressive infection-triggered inflammatory immune response that leads to over 2.9 million neonatal and pediatric deaths worldwide each year. Delays in recognition and treatment increase morbidity and mortality risk. Although predictive models have the potential to improve time to diagnosis and patient outcomes, developing these models for pediatric patients remains challenging. The integration of these tools into clinical practice requires good communication among team members, a solid provider foundation for medical decision-making, and cultural acceptance of machine learning in the clinical space. Future models should focus not only on mortality and in-hospital morbidity, but also on other meaningful measures, such as quality of life.

Keywords: Pediatric Sepsis · Machine Learning · Sepsis Prediction Models

1 Panel - Sepsis: Current Practices and Opportunities for Artificial Intelligence (AI) Applications

Sepsis is an infection-triggered inflammatory immune response [1]. It manifests as a progressive entity, beginning with tachycardia, fever, tachypnea, and hypotension, and in some cases evolution to multi-organ dysfunction and death [2]. Sepsis is responsible for over 2.9 million neonatal and pediatric deaths worldwide each year [3]. The current treatment strategy for sepsis is limited to antimicrobials and supportive care. Delays in recognition and treatment increase morbidity and mortality risk. However, its initial non-specific presentation and subtle progression can make timely diagnosis challenging. Recent research has focused on predictive computer models as potential tools to improve time to diagnosis and patient outcomes. In the adult population, several machine learning models for sepsis prediction have showed promise, including Conformal Multidimensional Prediction of Sepsis Risk (COMPOSER) [4], Sepsis Early Risk Assessment (SERA) [5], and the first FDA approved tool, Sepsis ImmunoScore (Prenosis, Chicago, IL, USA). Nonetheless, there are several challenges to the development of similar models for pediatric patients.

Poor outcomes in sepsis often result from delayed recognition and missed opportunities to intervene early before the disease progresses [1, 2, 6, 7]. Current pediatric

L. Ehwerhemuepha et al. (Eds.): IPLDSC 2024, CCIS 2386, pp. 81–83, 2025.
https://doi.org/10.1007/978-3-031-88346-0

sepsis alert tools are reactive, rather than predictive. Prediction allows for quicker implementation of diagnostic work-up, vascular access, and antibiotic initiation, which may reduce the risk of progression to multi-organ failure and death [2]. Machine learning allows for real time, continuous assessment of large amounts patient data, including laboratory and imaging studies, progress notes, and vital signs. Future models could also include genetic variants and biomarkers. Machine learning allows for a dynamic tool that will continue to evolve with additional cases over time [8]. The automated processing of large data sets could decrease provider cognitive burden and allow for better resource allocation of procedures and invasive monitoring [2]. This would be especially important during high census periods or when provider coverage is limited, such as during night or weekend shifts [2].

Although several sepsis warning systems exist in pediatric healthcare, they are too sensitive and lack specificity [2, 6, 7]. Frequent alarms for well-appearing patients who are not septic leads to alarm fatigue, rendering warning systems less effective [6]. These systems fall short because merely defining sepsis has been a challenge historically in the pediatric population. The 2005 International Pediatric Sepsis Consensus Conference definition of sepsis has been critiqued for its inadequate specificity and inability to predict multiorgan dysfunction or mortality [9]. More recently, the introduction of the Phoenix sepsis criteria in 2024 provides an evidence-based definition of sepsis that may improve the specificity of machine learning tools moving forward [9, 10]. Several pediatric institutions are currently developing machine learning models for sepsis prediction in the emergency department [2, 8], inpatient ward [6, 8], and intensive care unit [7].

Advances in predictive technology require a parallel strengthening of clinician judgement, especially in trainees [2, 8]. Machine learning models should enhance, rather than replace, provider decision making [2]. At times, it may be appropriate for a provider to decline a model's recommendation based on a particular clinical scenario. Conversely, providers must also take care not to dismiss model alerts without careful discretion. Ideally, a predictive tool will alert a provider before a child has reached multi-organ failure [7]. Providers may be prompted to treat well-appearing patients more proactively, before more overt signs and symptoms become apparent [8]. The integration of these tools into clinical practice requires good communication amongst team members, a solid provider foundation for medical decision making, and cultural acceptance of machine learning in the clinical space [2, 8].

With the promises of pediatric sepsis prediction models come unique challenges including social and ethical considerations. Many patients with sepsis who survive to discharge from the intensive care unit, experience a reduced quality of life [11]. From adjusting to new technology dependence to decreased performance scores, the social impacts of sepsis can develop and persist long after discharge [11]. Although reducing mortality and severe multi-organ dysfunction is an early goal for pediatric sepsis tools, other meaningful outcomes such as quality of life, should also be considered in future models [11]. Finally, it is important to include a diverse population in model development and training, in order to minimize bias [7].

Acknowledgements. A panel titled "Sepsis: Current Practices and Opportunities for Artificial Intelligence (AI) Applications" was held at the Pediatric and Lifespan Data Science Conference on May 23, 2024, in Anaheim, California, USA to discuss the future of predictive computer models in pediatric sepsis. We present highlights and primary themes from this discussion. The panel included the following speakers, whose ideas are represented here.

Moderator: Sandip Godambe, MD, PhD, MBA[1,2]

Speakers: Raina Paul, MD [1,2], Rachel Marano, MD[3,4], Robert B. Kelly, MD, FAAP [1,2], Robert Sepanski, MS [5,6], Elizabeth Killien, MD, MPH [7,8]

[1] Children's Hospital Orange County
[2] University of California Irvine
[3] Rady Children's Hospital
[4] University of California San Diego
[5] Children's Hospital of the King's Daughters
[6] Eastern Virginia Medical School
[7] Seattle Children's Hospital
[8] University of Washington School of Medicine

Disclosure of Interests. The authors have no relevant disclosures or conflicts of interest.

References

1. Godambe, S.: Sepsis: current practices and opportunities for AI applications. In: International Pediatric and Lifespan Data Science Conference, Anaheim, CA, USA (2024)
2. Paul, R.: AI for sepsis prediction in the emergency department. In: International Pediatric and Lifespan Data Science Conference, Anaheim, CA, USA (2024)
3. Global report on the epidemiology and burden of sepsis: current evidence, identifying gaps and future directions. World Health Organization (2020)
4. Shashikumar, S.P., Wardi, G., Malhotra, A., et al.: Artificial intelligence sepsis prediction algorithm learns to say "I don't know". npj Digit. Med. **4**, 134 (2021). https://doi.org/10. 1038/s41746-021-00504-6
5. Goh, K.H., et al.: Artificial intelligence in sepsis early prediction and diagnosis using unstructured data in healthcare. Nat. Commun. **12**, 711 (2021). https://doi.org/10.1038/ s41467-021-20910-4
6. Marano, R.: Pediatric sepsis in the inpatient setting. In: International Pediatric and Lifespan Data Science Conference, Anaheim, CA, USA (2024)
7. Kelly, R.: Creating a machine learning model for earlier prediction of sepsis in the pediatric intensive care unit. In: International Pediatric and Lifespan Data Science Conference, Anaheim, CA, USA (2024)
8. Sepanski, R.: Sepsis: current practices and opportunities for artificial intelligence applications. In: International Pediatric and Lifespan Data Science Conference, Anaheim, CA, USA (2024)
9. Sanchez-Pinto, L.N., et al.: Development and validation of the phoenix criteria for pediatric sepsis and septic shock. JAMA. **331**, 675–686 (2024). https://doi.org/10.1001/jama.2024. 0196
10. Schlapbach, L.J., et al.: International consensus criteria for pediatric sepsis and septic shock. JAMA. **331**, 665–674 (2024). https://doi.org/10.1001/jama.2024.0179
11. Killien, E.: Long-term outcomes among children surviving sepsis. In: International Pediatric and Lifespan Data Science Conference, Anaheim, CA, USA (2024)

Real-World Electronic Health Record Data for Research

Dena Jaffe[1], Jeffery Thompson[2], Joan Devin[3], Nik Koscielniak[4],
Rebecca Rosen[5], and Mark Hoffman[6(✉)]

[1] Oracle Health, Jerusalem, Israel
[2] Medical Center, University of Kansas, Kansas City, KS, USA
[3] Irish Medicines in Pregnancy Services, The Rotunda Hospital, Dublin, Ireland
[4] Patient-Centered Outcomes Research Institute (PCORI), Washington, DC, USA
[5] Eunice Kennedy Shriver National Institute of Child Health and Human Development (NICHD), National Institutes of Health (NIH), Maryland, USA
[6] Children's Mercy Kansas City, Kansas City, MO, USA
Mhoffman@cmh.edu

Abstract. This is a brief summary of the panel on Real-World Electronic Health Record Data for Research at the Inaugural International Pediatric and Lifespan Data Science Conference held by the Children's Hospital of Orange County at The Westin Anaheim Resort, California, USA.

Keywords: Electronic Health Records · Real-World Data

1 Introduction

Electronic health record (EHR) data is captured during the delivery of patient care and represents "real-world data" (RWD) describing clinical practice and decision-making. The volume of data available is much greater than that available through historic modes of performing clinical research (surveys, randomized clinical trials (RCTs)). Unfiltered EHR data can reveal patterns in care that lead to optimal outcomes or can reveal decisions that are not aligned with best practices [1, 2]. RWD has been discussed as an alternative or complement to RCTs and has been applied to a growing number of medication and device approvals [3]. During a recent panel discussion at the first annual International Pediatric and Lifespan Data Science conference, a group of experts convened to discuss the use of real-world EHR data for research. They shared modes of working with EHR data, a variety of opportunities related to EHR RWD and challenges in working with this data.

2 Modes of RWD Research

Research with RWD is most often performed in one of three modes – the use of an institutional data warehouse, multisite federated network and multisite aggregated data (Fig. 1).

© The Author(s) 2025
L. Ehwerhemuepha et al. (Eds.): IPLDSC 2024, CCIS 2386, pp. 84–88, 2025.
https://doi.org/10.1007/978-3-031-88346-0

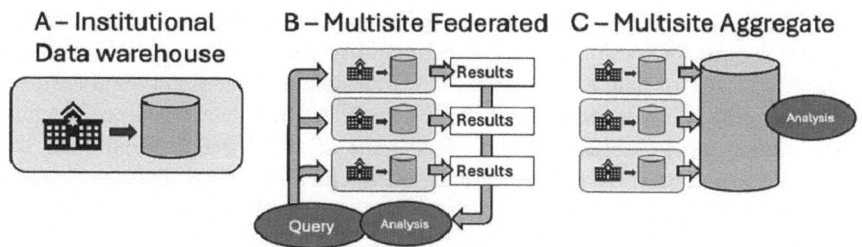

Fig. 1. Modes of Real-World Data Research

Institutional Data Warehouse: Most healthcare providers in the United States now use an EHR system, as do those in many other countries. One level of RWD research is to query local EHR data, seeking evidence of patterns within a single healthcare entity. For example, the University of Kansas uses their in-house developed Curated Cancer Clinical Outcomes Database (C3OD) to query their local data and has investigated disparities for cancer care in rural populations using this approach [4, 5]. The Rotunda Hospital in Ireland has a long history of formally documented medical records dating to 1787 and has used an EHR, the Maternal and Newborn Clinical Management System (MN-CMS), since 2017.

The Rotunda is one of four maternity hospitals that use MN-CMS and offers an example of the potential for national EHR analysis related to a clinical specialty. MN-CMS covers much of Ireland, including 40% of all births in Ireland (soon to be 70%) and providing 6–8 years of longitudinal data to approximately 3000 users. Data from the MN-CMS has been used to investigate venous thromboembolism (VTE) risk, medication errors, postpartum hemorrhage risk and prescribing trends for women of childbearing potential in individual sites. Researchers at the Rotunda Hospital used MN-CMS data to identify 84 "near-miss" medication errors [6].

Multisite Federated: The next level of EHR RWD research is the use of federated multi-institutional data for all care, regardless of specialty. One exemplary multi-site federated research network is PCORnet®, the National Patient-Centered Clinical Research Network, which is primarily funded by the Patient-Centered Outcomes Research Institute (PCORI) [7]. PCORnet is a large "network of networks" that seeks to efficiently enable national-scale health research, particularly patient-centered comparative clinical effectiveness research (CER). PCORnet has been used for over 45 national patient-centered PCORnet® Studies since 2020. While there are other multi-site research networks (e.g., Healthcare Systems Research Network), PCORnet is unique for many reasons, notably its focus on patient-centeredness in all facets of the network. PCORnet comprises a Coordinating Center and eight Clinical Research Networks (CRNs) which are groups of diverse healthcare institutions across the U.S. Collectively, the CRNs comprise 78 data-contributing partners with over 13,000 clinical sites, from large academic health centers to local community clinics, connected to more than 45 million unique U.S. patients annually, which includes nearly 13 million pediatric patients [8]. Each PCORnet data contributing partner stores a version of their clinical data in the PCORnet® Common Data Model (CDM). In this distributed network, the data stay behind the institutional firewall of each partner, protected under the Health Insurance Portability and Accountability Act of 1996 (HIPAA). Partners manage the transfer of data to the CRNs, the Coordinating Center and data requestors. As a public utility, any investigator can leverage PCORnet data resources for funded research studies or feasibility queries. A benefit of the federated approach is the retention of local control by PCORnet sites in how their site-level data are shared and used for research.

Multisite Aggregated: As an alternative to federated data, aggregate EHR data resources are offered by two large EHR vendors – Oracle and Epic. Contributing organizations enter into a data sharing agreement with their vendor and then regularly send data to the vendor where it is merged into a massive, HIPAA-compliant, data resource. Oracle has operated systems providing this capability for more than 20 years and aggregates data from more than 140 non-affiliated US health systems, including many smaller organizations. The Oracle EHR RWD platform is a foundational component of their Oracle Health Learning Health Network [9]. Epic offers their Cosmos resource. Cosmos began as a federated model and is transitioning to a true aggregate data platform. Cosmos offers a user-friendly front-end for performing queries against the aggregate data [10]. Both Oracle EHRRWD and Cosmos include data from more than 120 million US patients. The benefits of EHR-vendor provided aggregate resources are speed to query and reduced effort to participate. However, contributors are generally not able to monitor specific queries that include their data and access is generally limited to contributing organizations.

3   Opportunities and Challenges

RWD analysis offers many opportunities in research. Significantly, it represents clinical reality and as such, is useful for identifying and characterizing gaps in care, health equity concerns, and identifying opportunities to improve the consistency and quality of care. RWD also offers opportunities to ascertain subtle patterns in clinical outcomes. RWD enables researchers to evaluate off-label use of medications as a precursor to formal review. Privacy-preserving record linkage (PPRL) technologies enable the linkage of patient data across organizations, enabling longitudinal analysis of patient populations. For example, the FDA-sponsored Sentinel Initiative has used data linking to support pharmacoepidemiologic studies [11].

RWD research also entails many challenges. Use of data standards can vary within and across organizations. In the US, the lack of a consistent national health identifier makes it difficult to link data across disparate sources. Missing data in EHR systems can reflect workflow variation ("missing by design"), data loss in transition between the source system and the analysis platform, or differences in implementation [12]. Ensuring adherence to privacy policies, including HIPAA and the European General Data Protection Regulation (GDPR) is critical. The lack of inclusion of persons from under-represented communities in RWD resources reflects deeper issues in health access but has significant impact on the analyses performed using these resources. The use of PPRL to link data across organizations requires adherence to governance-associated requirements that arise from regulations, policies, organizations, and patients [13]. PPRL offers the important opportunity to connect lifespan data for patients who may have received care in a standalone pediatric facility as children and now receive care in separate organizations as adults. Data sharing promotes research reproducibility and equitable access. The 2023 NIH Policy for Data Management and Sharing defines data sharing as "The act of making scientific data available for use by others (e.g., the larger research community, institutions, the broader public), for example, via an established repository" [14]. NIH published supplemental guidance on protecting research participant privacy when sharing data through the use of controlled access data repositories [15]. For example, the NICHD Clinical Trials Networks share data through the Data and Specimen Hub (DASH) [16], As allowed by data use agreements, data sharing processes could be incorporated into each of the RWD research modes described here.

The panelists identified future directions of shared interest. These include continued progress toward the effective and collaborative governance of RWD resources and development of ontologies that enhance the structure of data. There was strong interest in enabling the connection of data across the lifespan of a patient. For example, when a child becomes an adult, data from a stand-alone pediatric hospital may not be connected to data generated later in their life. The panel also expressed interest in seeking ways to use the analysis of RWD to inform providers at the point of care.

4 Conclusion

EHR systems generate massive amounts of data as a byproduct of delivering patient care. Unfiltered EHR data provides a strong example of "real world data" as it represents care patterns in a variety of settings. Local analysis of this data stored in a data warehouse can generate insights that inform research and quality improvement. Analysis of EHR data from disparate sites, whether through a federated model or through an aggregate warehouse, can enable researchers to compare care across non-affiliated organizations. While there are significant opportunities to use EHR RWD for epidemiology and health disparities; there are also considerable challenges of standardization, handling missing data, and reconciling system-level variation.

Acknowledgements. The authors wish to acknowledge the organizers of the First Annual International Pediatric and Lifespan Data Science Conference, especially Dr. Louis Ehwerhemuepha and Aline Rohloff.

Disclosure of Interests. The authors have no competing interests to declare that are relevant to the content of this article.

References

1. Connelly, M., Glynn, E.F., Hoffman, M.A., Bickel, J.: Rates and predictors of using opioids in the emergency department to treat migraine in adolescents and young adults. Pediatr. Emerg. Care **37**, e981–e987 (2019)
2. Sivasankar, S., Cheng, A.L., Lubin, I.M., Lankachandra, K., Hoffman, M.A.: Use of large scale EHR data to evaluate A1c utilization among sickle cell disease patients. BMC Med. Inform. Decis. Mak. **21**(1), 268. (2021). https://doi.org/10.1186/s12911-021-01632-5
3. Purpura, C.A., Garry, E.M., Honig, N., Case, A., Rassen, J.A.: The role of real-world evidence in FDA-approved new drug and biologics license applications. Clin. Pharmacol. Ther. **111**(1), 135–144 (2022)
4. Thompson, J.A., et al.: The need to study rural cancer outcome disparities at the local level: a retrospective cohort study in Kansas and Missouri. BMC Public Health **21**(1), 2154. (2021). https://doi.org/10.1186/s12889-021-12190-w
5. Mudaranthakam, D.P., et al.: A curated cancer clinical outcomes database (C3OD) for accelerating patient recruitment in cancer clinical trials. JAMIA Open. **1**(2), 166–171 (2018)
6. Devin, J., Cullinan, S., Looi, C., Cleary, B.J.: Identification of prescribing errors in an electronic health record using a retract-and-reorder tool: a pilot study. J. Patient Saf. **18**(7), e1076–e1082 (2022)
7. Fleurence, R.L., et al.: Launching PCORnet, a national patient-centered clinical research network. J. Am. Med. Inform. Assoc. JAMIA **21**(4), 578–582 (2014)
8. PCORnet: Characteristics of the pediatric population across clinical research networks participating in PCORnet: PCORnet (2024). https://pcornet.org/wp-content/uploads/2024/09/Public_Query_Report_Pediatric_PCORnet_Query_Final.pdf
9. Ehwerhemuepha, L., et al.: Cerner real-world data (CRWD) - A de-identified multicenter electronic health records database. Data Brief **42**, 108120 (2022)
10. Tarabichi, Y., et al.: The cosmos collaborative: a vendor-facilitated electronic health record data aggregation platform. ACI open. **5**(1), e36–e46 (2021)
11. Sentinel: Inclusion of Semi-Structured and Unstructured Electronic Health Record (EHR) Data in Confounding Adjustment and Outcome Ascertainment (2024). https://www.sentinelinitiative.org/methods-data-tools/methods/inclusion-semi-structured-and-unstructured-electronic-health-record-ehr
12. Glynn, E.F., Hoffman, M.A.: Heterogeneity introduced by EHR system implementation in a de-identified data resource from 100 non-affiliated organizations. JAMIA Open. **2**(4), 554–561 (2019)
13. ODSS N: Record Linkage Implementation Checklist: NICHD (2024). https://www.nichd.nih.gov/sites/default/files/inline-files/Record_Linkage_Implementation_Checklist.pdf
14. NIH: Final NIH Policy for Data Management and Sharing (2023). https://grants.nih.gov/grants/guide/notice-files/NOT-OD-21-013.html
15. NIH: Supplemental Information to the NIH Policy for Data Management and Sharing: Protecting Privacy When Sharing Human Research Participant Data (2022). https://grants.nih.gov/grants/guide/notice-files/NOT-OD-22-213.html
16. Hazra, R., et al.: DASH, the data and specimen hub of the National Institute of Child Health and Human Development. Sci. Data **5**, 180046 (2018)

Author Index

L. Ehwerhemuepha et al. (Eds.): IPLDSC 2024, CCIS 2386, p. 89, 2025.
https://doi.org/10.1007/978-3-031-88346-0